CANDACE
PERT

CANDACE PERT

*Genius, Greed, and Madness
in the World of Science*

PAMELA RYCKMAN

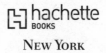

NEW YORK

Hachette Books
Hachette Book Group
1290 Avenue of the Americas
New York, NY 10104
HachetteBooks.com
Twitter.com/HachetteBooks
Instagram.com/HachetteBooks

First Edition: November 2023

Published by Hachette Books, an imprint of Hachette Book Group, Inc. The Hachette Books name and logo is a trademark of the Hachette Book Group.

The Hachette Speakers Bureau provides a wide range of authors for speaking events. To find out more, go to hachettespeakersbureau.com or email HachetteSpeakers@hbgusa.com.

Books by Hachette Books may be purchased in bulk for business, educational, or promotional use. For information, please contact your local bookseller or Hachette Book Group Special Markets Department at special.markets@hbgusa.com.

The publisher is not responsible for websites (or their content) that are not owned by the publisher.

Print book interior design by Linda Mark.

Library of Congress Cataloging-in-Publication Data
Names: Ryckman, Pamela, author.
Title: Candace Pert: genius, greed, and madness in the world of science / Pamela Ryckman.
Description: First edition. | New York, NY : Hachette Books, 2023. | Includes bibliographical references.
Identifiers: LCCN 2023017584 | ISBN 9780306831461 (hardcover) | ISBN 9780306831485 (ebook)
Subjects: LCSH: Pert, Candace B., 1946-2013. | Psychopharmacologists—United States—Biography. | Integrative medicine—United States—Biography. | Feminists—United States—Biography.
Classification: LCC RC464.P49 R93 2023 | DDC 616.89/18092—dc23/eng/20230705
LC record available at https://lccn.loc.gov/2023017584

ISBNs: 978-0-306-83146-1 (hardcover); 978-0-306-83148-5 (ebook)

Printed in the United States of America

LSC-C

Printing 1, 2023

For Candace, may you rest in peace

CONTENTS

Contents

INTRODUCTION

You must have chaos within you
to give birth to a dancing star.

—Friedrich Nietzsche

C ANDACE BEEBE PERT STOOD AT THE DAWN OF THREE REVOLUTIONS: THE WOM-
en's movement, psychopharmacology, and integrative health. A scientific prodigy, she was thirty years ahead of her time, preaching a
holistic approach to healthcare and medicine long before yoga hit the
mainstream and "wellness" took root in our vernacular. As mother of
the mind-body revolution, Candace launched a paradigm shift—but
not without a fight.

I read *Molecules of Emotion*, Candace's provocative memoir and
exposé of the cutthroat scientific establishment, almost twenty years
after its 1997 publication, yet still it packed a punch. I marveled that
the same woman who'd discovered the opiate receptor in 1972 as a
twenty-six-year-old graduate student had also proved the mind-body
link *and* created Peptide T, the underground AIDS drug featured in
the film *Dallas Buyers Club*. As daily headlines announced the opioid

1

crisis's devastating toll, Candace's work felt surprisingly relevant, so I devoured her second book, *Everything You Need to Know to Feel Go(o)d*, and watched her appearances on *Larry King Live* and Bill Moyers's *Healing and the Mind* as well as in the 2004 documentary *What the Bleep Do We Know?*, which gained a cult following and increased her renown.

Candace's interdisciplinary insights related neuroscience, pharmacology, immunology, and virology at a time when most scientists and doctors never looked beyond the narrow confines of their specialties. In the early 1980s she demonstrated that, rather than being a control center, the brain works together with the endocrine, immune, and gastrointestinal systems to produce the thoughts and emotions that define our reality. Contrary to most neuropharmacologists at the time, she lobbied for natural solutions, warning that when it comes to prescription drugs, "less is best." She counseled that our minds could be used to heal our bodies, and vice versa.

Though Candace's views were seen as radical and went largely unsupported during her tenure as chief of brain biochemistry at the National Institute of Mental Health (NIMH), a subsidiary of the National Institutes of Health (NIH), her studies formed the basis of the now booming field of embodied cognition. Today, scientists across the globe continue to monitor the interconnections between thoughts and emotions, emphasizing how integral our feelings are to healing. Bessel van der Kolk, a psychiatrist who has spent thirty years studying trauma and has received grants from both the NIMH and the National Center for Complementary and Integrative Health (NCCIH), affirms Candace's findings that psychology and physiology are intertwined. In his bestselling book *The Body Keeps the Score: Brain, Mind, and Body in the Healing of Trauma*, he explains how trauma produces physiological changes such as recalibrating the brain's alarm system.

Given that one in ten Americans now takes antidepressants and half a million children in the United States are prescribed antipsychotics, van der Kolk echoes Candace when he writes that "the drug revolution that started out with so much promise may in the end have done as much harm as good." He also posits that psychiatric medications often mask symptoms while leaving the underlying causes of trauma untreated. And, because we now know that the brain has plasticity, as it is wired by experiences rather than genes, van der Kolk instead advocates techniques Candace espoused decades ago, such as meditation, yoga, biofeedback, theater, and eye movement desensitization and reprocessing (EMDR), to reprogram our brains at the cellular level.

Likewise, Lisa Feldman Barrett, who is among the top 1 percent of most-cited scientists in the world for her research in psychology and neuroscience, says that Candace's discoveries are built into the fabric of her work. "So much of what she wrote about are not hypotheses anymore; they're ground assumptions, assumed to be fact, to the extent that they're not even attached to her name," says Barrett, a University Distinguished Professor of Psychology at Northeastern University. "I walk in this woman's shoes. I stand on her shoulders." In her 2017 book *How Emotions Are Made: The Secret Life of the Brain*, Barrett refines Candace's findings to explain that emotions are not emitted from a specific part of the brain, nor do they have a biological fingerprint. Rather, we construct our emotions spontaneously, becoming "architects of our own experience." Our experiences are the amalgam of a complex dance between brain and body, which therefore must be studied and treated holistically.

Following Candace's lead, Barrett notes that stress and trauma may cause the misallocation of energy and resources assigned to various physiological functions, which can lead to anything from chronic pain to heart disease and cancer. Increasingly, scientists also acknowledge that illnesses previously dismissed as mental disorders (e.g., anxiety, depression, and even autism) have roots in the physical, as inflammation results from persistent "misbudgeting." "New discoveries about the nervous system are dissolving the sacred boundary between what we think of as physical and mental illness," Barrett reports, confirming Candace's insights.

However, while Candace focused mainly on chemical communication, Barrett makes a case for wiring. "She was thinking about the brain as a bag of chemicals, but it's not only a bag of chemicals. . . . There's also electrical communication, which is faster and more expensive, and she doesn't talk about it. It's not that this is more true, it's just also true," Barrett says. "From my perspective, that was an oversight, but I'm saying this in 2022. I wouldn't expect her to have had the whole picture."

During Candace's lifetime, her message often fell on deaf ears, for science is resistant to change and original ideas are slow to take root. As Naomi Oreskes asserts in her 2019 book *Why Trust Science?*, the field is based on consensus rather than universal truths. When scientists with varying backgrounds and points of view arrive at the same conclusions through observation and analysis, consensus is born. Then, even "absolutes" can change. Ideally, a scientist retains a beginner's mind throughout her career, remaining open to new data even when they contradict earlier findings. The profession requires that one modifies interpretations, formulates new hypotheses, and tests them. If, however, a researcher becomes mired in certain dogma, she ceases to practice science and begins practicing religion.

Regardless, as the saying goes, "science proceeds one funeral at a time," and researchers who've built their careers defending a worldview often champion their beliefs even in the face of conflicting evidence. Only after they die or their influence wanes do the edicts of a new generation take hold. Candace died before her perspective was fully embraced by the scientific establishment, but she'd pioneered a course of study that did not previously exist. "In neuroscience, biology, pharmacology, and psychology, people are taking mind-body connections very seriously," Barrett says. "That's what a scientist's true legacy is. It's not just to publish papers; it's to seed the field so that the next generation of scientists can carry forward ideas and do miraculous things."

Indeed, Candace was a visionary. What's more, she was a character in the truest sense of the word, a lightning rod for trouble. She had an obsessive quality that was contagious, and during hundreds of hours of interviews with her family, friends, and colleagues, I've found one common thread: no one can let her go.

Initially I set my sights on making a film about her life and approached her widower, Michael Ruff, in 2016 to secure the rights to her memoir. However, because it was published twenty-five years ago and Candace passed away in 2013, I also sought Michael's help facilitating interviews with associates who might fill in the gaps. How did her story end?

I was eager to know what became of Candace, but the more I researched, the more things didn't add up. I discovered that, in writing *Molecules of Emotion*, she had not only presented herself in a flattering light, as memoirists are wont to do, but also twisted the truth. Her existence was more complex than she let on, and her moral compass more compromised. Throughout her life, Candace was besieged by bloodsuckers keen to profit from her brilliance, until she too succumbed to greed.

Yes, Candace was a genius whose breakthroughs shaped history. But while working as a seeker and sage merging science with spirituality, she'd become the ultimate wounded healer, tainted by hubris, consumed by demons, and riddled with regret. I knew that, for science, Candace had ventured to the edge, but how far would she go in the name of healing?

CHAPTER ONE

EUREKA!

"**H**OLD STILL, YOU FUCKIN' RAT!"

Candace Pert sat in her underwear on the bathroom floor, her hairy legs crossed and a thin cigarillo dangling from her lips. Her four-year-old son, Evan, and his teenage babysitter, Deborah Stokes, stood rapt as she struggled to inject a squirming rodent. She edged the needle closer, piercing its skin before tossing it back in its cage. Once dressed, she'd call morgues for cadavers before driving to her lab to behead hamsters, gouging out and blending their brains into a frothy soup for study.

"I'd never known anyone like her," Stokes says. Candace lived for science.

In 1971, she was less than a year into her graduate studies in neuro-pharmacology at Johns Hopkins University School of Medicine, where she had the good fortune to train under Solomon Snyder, a dazzling "golden boy" of the medical establishment who was, at age thirty-one, the university's youngest full professor. As a neuropharmacologist and psychiatrist running the PhD program, Snyder was pursuing exactly what Candace longed to do: combine the examination of brain chemistry with an analysis of human behavior for a real-world application of drugs. Better still, he was part of a scientific dynasty that linked the profession's best and brightest, a lineage that electrified their field.

Research science follows an apprenticeship model akin to artists and architects, and luminaries often trace lines of mentorship back to early trailblazers. Wisdom and knowledge filter through generations by both instruction and osmosis, and mentors serve as benefactors invested in the long-term success of their progeny. Lab chiefs call in favors to secure plum positions for protégés, seeding a global network of trusted comrades on whom to call for the duration of each member's career. Like an exclusive old boys' club or Ivy League university, the whole is greater than the sum of its parts, and membership has privileges.

In science, it is said that 90 percent of groundbreaking discoveries are made by a select 10 percent of investigators, and this elite cohort just happens to be the same web of scientists descended from pioneers. Remarkably, researchers attempting to isolate the distinguishing traits of Nobel Prize winners have been surprised to find that—rather than IQ, parental engagement, alma mater, or socioeconomic status—one's mentor or scientific lineage is the determining factor, as at least half of all scientific Nobel laureates studied and trained under other Nobel laureates. As a result, a researcher's early pedigree is defined as much by her "genealogy" as by her personal achievements.

Candace knew that in joining Sol Snyder's lab, she was being adopted into a scientific royal family, receiving keys to the kingdom. Snyder was in constant contact with his revered mentor, Julius Axelrod, who had won the Nobel Prize just a year before for his work on the release, reuptake, and storage of catecholamine neurotransmitters (i.e., dopamine, norepinephrine [noradrenaline], and epinephrine [adrenaline]) in the brain, which had revealed how the body processes and regulates these chemical messengers. And Axelrod, for whom Snyder had worked as a research associate from 1963 to 1965, had trained under Bernard Beryl "Steve" Brodie, the veritable father of modern neuro-pharmacology, the study of how drugs impact the nervous system to influence behavior. Brodie was credited with originating an entire field with his leading-edge demonstration of how the human body interacts with and transforms the chemicals it absorbs.

Now Snyder was grooming Candace in the freewheeling, intuitive approach to science that he had learned from Axelrod, who had learned it from Brodie. Brodie descendants focused on "hot science," or big, bold leaps that addressed grand questions of the day. These researchers reveled in probing the great unknown, approaching science with the wonder of children. Fancying themselves noble explorers, they stressed that existing scientific literature described only what was known, not what had yet to be found. Instead of diligently consulting journals, they brainstormed with peers, batting around ideas to unearth some new kernel of truth, some technique or data that might be applied in one's own lab. For this lot, science was a high-stakes, exuberant adventure filled with trailblazing discovery that blended logic with instinct and artistry to unlock the mysteries of life.

Brodie stock remained flexible. They strove to see the "big pic-ture," investigating how a domain related to other fields. Theirs was an adrenaline-fueled, entrepreneurial approach to science in which researchers took risks, failed, and recovered quickly. They were taught to speculate freely and question authority or accepted wisdom. Crack-ling with new ideas, they followed hunches and kept their eyes peeled for results that seemed peculiar or unique, adjusting experiments to suit penetrating observations as they arose. Like jazz musicians, they riffed and extrapolated, building upon each other's thoughts. No need to chart a course at the outset, they said, but rather follow the tune and delight in the journey. It was bound to lead somewhere great.

Brodie's "scientific family" was also marked by aggressive ambition, as members "skimmed the cream," capitalizing on the ponderous work of others to leapfrog to crucial innovations. Unlike other scientists who made tiny inroads by plodding through detailed assays, or analyses of substances and their concentrations, this group would "take a flier on it," designing simple, quick-and-dirty experiments that granted enough information to know whether an idea held promise. Why spend weeks or months in a library mapping out an assay when a few hours in a lab would yield the same answer?

If early experiments augured well, Brodie's researchers followed the meticulous path with appropriate controls. If not, they jumped to the next conjecture. Doing so eschewed tedium and ensured that no one got bogged down in low-impact trials. Instead, they'd plant seeds to see what sprouted, take shortcuts to meaningful insights, and scoop rivals to clinch a final victory or prize. Perhaps their methods were unorthodox, but they produced astounding results.

Thus, Sol Snyder's fiefdom at Hopkins pulsed with his pupils' thirst to prevail. If science was a game to be won, then Snyder was grandmaster, goading mentees to spar not only with other labs but also with each other, as each student angled for his attention and praise. Presiding over at least a dozen projects (three or four times as many as other lab chiefs), Snyder was kinetic, always in motion, assessing new ground and guiding acolytes who flew in formation. Even his features, pointed and birdlike, suggested a capacity to see from a great distance, home in on a target, and dive in for the kill.

When Candace arrived in Snyder's lab as one of a select eight to ten postdoctoral fellows, PhD students, and MD-PhD students, the "neurosciences" were just being defined. Working at the crossroads of psychiatry, biochemistry, neurology, and pharmacology, Snyder was fixated on identifying new neurotransmitters, or chemicals secreted in the brain that were thought to convey information to direct the body's actions and emotions. He aimed to probe the chemistry of the brain to understand the biological basis of mental illness and then devise treatments.

"Sol knew that the work being done in his lab was at the center of a revolution and communicating this to his students was part of his charisma," Candace writes in her memoir, *Molecules of Emotion*. "He had a way of letting us know we were on the cutting edge, caught up in a grand and glorious gamble, which, if we won, would make us all stars."

Candace loved gleaning meaning from oceans of data. But initially she'd struggled with the workload at Hopkins and had quickly earned a reputation as exuberant yet impatient and somewhat sloppy. So, on the advice of the department's senior faculty, Snyder devised for her a structured path toward a dissertation that seemed a surefire success. She was to refine the earlier findings of his postdoc Dr. Hank Yamamura, researching how the body regulates the production of acetylcholine, the first-discovered and most common neurotransmitter that was known to slow the heartbeat and impact memory circuits in the brain. While Snyder assumed Candace would jump at a "bread-and-butter" study, instead she balked at this humdrum task. Candace longed to solve complex riddles of her own, not play second fiddle to a postdoc.

For her graduate thesis, Candace sought a project that would set her apart from the crowd, one that addressed a real-world issue whose impact would be seen and felt. Such an opportunity appeared when, on June 17, 1971, President Richard Nixon declared a war on drugs. America's drug problem had been front-page news since the late 1960s, as "flower children" increasingly migrated from marijuana and LSD to amphetamines and heroin, the last an opioid made from morphine, which is produced in the seed pod of opium poppy plants. Across the nation, a spike in crime rates was increasingly blamed on an epidemic of addiction, and heroin use had spread to the white middle class. The press was riddled with stories of teenagers dying from overdoses, even decades before the current opioid crisis.

Moreover, an estimated 25 percent of the 270,000 American soldiers serving in Vietnam were hooked on a form of heroin that was far more potent than the version commonly available on American streets. Drug abuse of all sorts was said to be driving barbarous acts by American troops, including the 1968 My Lai massacre during which U.S. soldiers gang-raped, mutilated, and slaughtered between 347 and 504 South Vietnamese civilians, including infants and children. With reports of wasted, dispirited, and increasingly monstrous soldiers overseas, the American public was growing weary of this foreign war just as Nixon sought to escalate bombing in North Vietnam.

The president knew that taking credit for a decline in addiction and drug-related crime would bolster his case for reelection. Vowing to sweep junkies from American streets, Nixon established the Special Action Office for Drug Abuse Prevention to distribute federal funds for biomedical research to isolate and treat the causes of addiction. Dr. Jerome Jaffe, an eminent psychiatrist with extensive experience treating heroin addicts, was named the agency's "czar," affording heretofore unprecedented political acclaim to a physician.

For years Sol Snyder had known Jaffe as a comrade in arms, part of a small cadre of psychiatrists who, like himself, were interested less in psychoanalysis than in the biology of mental illness. When Snyder learned of Jaffe's appointment, he immediately offered to help. Admittedly, his intentions were far from selfless; Snyder saw an opportunity to further his personal goals by staking a claim to funds being appropriated by Congress. He knew that once scientists were able to pinpoint the cause of opiate addiction, they might find the source of other addictions such as alcohol and nicotine, or even develop a nonaddictive opiate that would alleviate the chronic pain suffered by millions. Here was a chance for Snyder to make his name.

Candace, in turn, had developed a fascination with opiates during the summer of 1970 after a horseback riding accident at Fort Sam in San Antonio, Texas. She'd moved there with her husband, Agu, an experimental psychologist who was fulfilling part of his military requirement, being trained as a Mobile Army Surgical Hospital (M.A.S.H.) unit commander in a three-month medical service course at a burn center for Vietnam veterans. To pass the time, Candace had taken riding lessons from a stern, aggressive colonel, and almost immediately she'd tumbled and injured her back, suffering a compression fracture of her first lumbar vertebra.

In the hospital, she'd been surrounded by soldiers just back from Vietnam, many of whom were addicted to heroin. When Candace received Demerol to ease her pain, she understood why. The drug transported her to a state of woozy bliss, and she spent much of that summer flat on her back, free from discomfort or distress about both her injury and her separation from Agu and their young son.

When she was lucid enough to read, Candace had called Snyder to ask how she might prepare for her upcoming graduate studies in neuropharmacology, and he'd recommended *Principles of Drug Action: The Basis of Pharmacology* by Avram Goldstein, Lewis Aronow, and S. M. Kalman. In this seminal text, Candace discovered the mechanism for the sublime sensation she'd experienced each time a nurse injected her with intramuscular morphine, and the reason she'd been tempted to abscond with extra doses upon departure. Candace never got hooked on the drug, but she craved an understanding of how opiates functioned. Though her back had healed by the time she began the PhD program at Hopkins, opiates remained fresh on her mind.

At that point, doctors and scientists knew that opiates worked on the brain, but they didn't know how. For centuries, physicians and poets alike had extolled the pain relief and euphoria caused by derivatives of the poppy plant. Modern researchers also observed that opiates depress breathing, suppress cough, trigger nausea, and constrict the pupils of the eyes. Yet no one had located the spot in the body that set off these changes. Where and how did opiates interact to initiate such diverse outcomes?

Logic dictated that for drugs to function in the body, they needed to adhere to receptors, or molecules that float on a cell's surface but have roots plunging deep inside. Receptors act as docking stations for drugs that fit into them like a key in a lock and initiate a chain of biochemical reactions. They are also specific, binding only to certain chemical keys, or ligands. The word "ligand" is derived from the Latin *ligo*, which means "to tie" or "to bind," and thus a ligand is a binding substance. Exogenous (external) drugs are ligands that mimic the body's endogenous (internal) hormones and neurotransmitters, faithfully targeting specific receptors to elicit a precise response.

The receptor concept was first proposed in the early twentieth century by Paul Ehrlich, the Nobel Prize–winning German physician and scientist who discovered salvarsan, the arsenic-based treatment for syphilis, and sketched schemas to illustrate how drugs might be recognized in the body. Until recently, however, no one had proved receptors' existence, though ample evidence pointed in their direction.

First, doctors had long been combatting overdoses with "antagonists," drugs known to reverse or block the effects of opiates. For instance, a shot of naloxone was known to prompt near-miraculous recovery in victims of heroin overdose, presumably because naloxone occupies the same receptors, thereby knocking off heroin or thwarting it from attaching. Next, researchers had observed that the effects of opiates increase with dose, but at a certain point they produce no additional response; saturation stood to reason, as there was presumably a finite number of each receptor in the body. Finally, scientists knew that opiates were stereospecific, meaning that on a molecular level they exist in mirror-image forms that are chemically identical except that one is "right-handed," while the other is "left-handed." Only the left-handed version of opiate drugs is effective, which indicates that the binding site is characterized by highly specific recognition.

Avram Goldstein, a pharmacology professor at Stanford, had devoted fifteen pages of *Principles of Drug Action* to explaining receptors and had been one of a mere handful of narcotic researchers committed to finding the opiate receptor in hopes of curing addiction. However, once the Nixon administration announced its war on drugs and allocated more than $6 million for research (the equivalent of $40 million today), labs nationwide had all the incentive they needed. The race was on.

During the summer of 1971, Snyder had taken copious notes at a lecture given by Goldstein following the publication of his coauthored paper "Stereospecific and Nonspecific Interactions of the Morphine Congener Levorphanol in Subcellular Fractions of Mouse Brain," which had recently appeared in the *Proceedings of the National Academy of Sciences*. While Goldstein's attempts to locate the opiate receptor had failed, his strategy was sound, so Snyder speculated that his methods could be refined for success. Like his legendary mentors, Snyder believed he could build upon Goldstein's foundation to "skim the cream." If finding the opiate receptor was the first step in eradicating chronic pain and drug dependence, then creating a nonaddictive opiate was surely the holy grail.

Once Candace learned that Snyder was securing grant money, she begged to abandon her dull acetylcholine assays to pursue this moonshot for her doctoral dissertation. "Now here was a goal I could easily imagine pursuing, a project worthy of my dreams, my ambitions, my aspirations," she writes. In the tradition of her esteemed scientific family, she would tackle one of the most pressing issues of her day.

Competition was fierce, but instead of deterring Candace, rivalry fueled her. While completing her required courses, she pored over Goldstein's paper and embarked on a two-month rotation with Pedro Cuatrecasas, a wunderkind endocrinologist and pharmacologist who, the previous year, had discovered the receptor for the hormone insulin, which is secreted by the pancreas and controls the body's blood sugar level and metabolism. In Cuatrecasas's lab, Candace learned a technique first employed in the 1950s: using radioactive chemical tracers to locate where a drug acts in the body. One of the drug's atoms is replaced with a radioactive isotope of the same element, and then the drug is blended in a test tube with homogenized tissue. The mixture is filtered under vacuum pressure to measure where the radioactive drug has bound to the tissue. To characterize the insulin receptor, Cuatrecasas had pioneered a rapid filtration method that would prove vital to Candace's subsequent work.

Candace and Snyder regularly compared notes, identifying Avram Goldstein's missteps and laboring to correct them. Meanwhile, she toiled long hours in the lab, relentlessly trying every variation of Goldstein's method. She monitored the ingredients in each day's mixture as well as other variables, switching drugs and modifying temperatures and incubation times. In this way, Candace's approach diverged from her mentors': far from flying by the seat of her pants, she was tenacious and steadfast, even dogged in pursuit—initially to no avail.

After six months of failed attempts, she had a lightning-bolt moment. Maybe the "hot" or radioactive dihydromorphine she'd been using in her experiments wasn't the right trace, or substance to track

toward an endpoint. Until now, she'd exclusively employed opiate agonists, or drugs that, upon binding with putative receptors, shift cellular activity. What if she tried antagonists instead? Candace had read
a paper by the English pharmacologist W. D. M. Paton that theorized
why agonists and antagonists function differently, and she'd learned
that certain antagonists are more potent than opiates. Perhaps this
meant that an antagonist would compete more aggressively for receptors, like sperm to an egg, and provide a clearer line to her target.

Candace's husband, Agu, was using the drug naloxone, a known
opiate antagonist, to counteract analgesia in test monkeys in his lab
at Edgewood Arsenal, the Maryland-based chemical warfare research
institute where he now worked. Perhaps if she was able to make naloxone radioactive or "hot," she could follow it straight to the bull's-eye.
Snyder, however, was unconvinced. The wisdom of his mentors dictated that when early efforts fail to yield evocative results, it is best
to move on. Plus, radioactive naloxone couldn't simply be ordered
from a catalogue; it had to be custom-made and, at $300 per unit, was
expensive. Candace appeared to have wasted half a year, and Snyder
couldn't afford to spend additional resources on her wild goose chase.
As her advisor, he had the responsibility of making sure she earned a
degree, and he insisted that Candace return to the more basic acetylcholine experiment he'd initially proposed. In short, Snyder was pulling the plug.

Candace griped and sulked before reluctantly acquiescing, but
secretly she hatched a plan. While Snyder was away at a conference,
she convinced Agu to acquire some cold, or nonradioactive, naloxone,
which she then sent to the Boston-based New England Nuclear Corporation, the go-to company for medical researchers, to be made radioactive. Because she lacked a radiation license, Candace either forged
an authorized user's signature or listed herself and somehow escaped

officials' scrutiny. Regardless, after retrieving her illicit parcel from Hopkins Radiation Control weeks later, she prepared to perform a clandestine assay on a Friday night, once Snyder and her lab mates had departed.

On the evening of October 22, 1972, just as she'd begun, Agu called to say that their babysitter was sick and couldn't retrieve their son Evan from his Montessori school. Quickly, Candace made a calculation: she'd need at least an hour to set up the experiment, which meant that she could dash to pick up Evan but would have to bring him back to the lab to finish in time. Yet how to sneak Evan past the guards, given the university's prohibitions against children near radioactive substances? She took a flier on it.

Once safely inside the lab, Candace gave Evan thirty-six vials to uncap while she hurried to transfer the brain membrane filters that were core to her experiment, using three variables for each cluster of twelve. The first group held pure radioactive ("hot") naloxone; the second, levorphanol, a powerful opiate, combined with hot naloxone; and the third, dextrophan, a non-opiate, combined with hot naloxone. She placed her test tubes in a counting machine and waited on pins and needles until Monday for results.

When Monday arrived, Candace raced early to the lab and opened a notebook to record her findings on a sheet of scientific graph paper. Slowly she copied numbers from the machine. When she found a low count of radiation in the tubes filled with levorphanol plus hot naloxone, it indicated that the two substances had competed to bind with the receptor and naloxone had lost. Meanwhile, tubes with dextrophan plus hot naloxone had high counts because, as a non-opiate, dextrophan could not bind to the opiate receptor. And tubes with only hot naloxone had the highest counts because the antagonist lacked any competition.

Candace shrieked with joy. This was exactly the outcome she'd desired, the stereospecific binding that researchers the world over were seeking. "O my god! It worked!" she wrote at the bottom of her protocol paper. "Will it continue to work? I bow to the great God of science!"

Later, Candace would dedicate her doctoral dissertation to her husband—"For Agu, who has given me love, Evan, encouragement, and naloxone"—but for now she savored this eureka flash. In finding the opiate receptor, she'd achieved the kind of breakthrough most scientists only dream about. Candace believed she'd taken the first step toward ending drug dependence, laying the groundwork for the creation of a nonaddictive opiate. She never could have imagined the nightmare she'd set in motion.

CHAPTER TWO

SHAINA MAIDEL

C ANDACE WAS DRIVEN FROM AN EARLY AGE, AND SHE RELISHED BEING A teacher's pet whose talent distinguished her from the pack. Flashing a ready smile and dark, hooded eyes that revealed her Eastern European heritage, she was always up for a challenge, quick to answer a question or act on a dare. "Some kids stand out," says Nancy Marriott, who befriended Candace in a Brownie troop in second grade. "Candace was a star, set for greatness from day one."

As the eldest of three sisters and the first grandchild in a fierce, close-knit matriarchy, she was also a leader at home. Candace's maternal grandfather, David Rosenberg, was descended from wealthy Lithuanian Jews who'd emigrated to the United States in the mid-nineteenth century, while his wife Rose's family had fled persecution in Ukraine. One of nine children, Rose was beautiful, vain, and proud of the advantageous match that enabled her to raise her daughters, Mildred and Lillian, with the help of servants in a grand home in Chester, Pennsylvania. That is, until the stock market crash of 1929.

While Rose was strict and selfish, David was a classic mensch, a compassionate property owner who'd been forced into bankruptcy and lost his own home after failing to collect rent from starving tenants, thus placing himself and his wife at the mercy of extended family. Rose grudgingly relocated to Atlantic City, New Jersey, to live in a cramped apartment behind a candy store and soda fountain David's brothers had purchased and that he would now manage. For a woman as status conscious as Rose, this fall from financial grace exacted a harsh toll, and her anger simmered at the surface.

Keen to restore her family's standing, she moved to orchestrate profitable marriages for her daughters and was devastated when Mildred fell in love and eloped with Bob Beebe, a penniless World War II veteran. Lithe and handsome with a brooding gaze, Bob was a sensitive artist and musician who had "cracked up" after his tour of duty as a medic cleaning up bodies in the South Pacific. He was being treated for "shell shock," or what is now called post-traumatic stress disorder (PTSD), at the hospital where Mildred worked. Each time a car backfired, Bob would dive under a bed, and later, when his daughters asked what he did during the war, Bob would say, "I hid."

While the Rosenbergs attended an Orthodox temple, Bob was a "goy" from a clan of Congregationalist ministers in New Britain, Connecticut. His father, Joseph, taught at The Hill School in Pennsylvania, while his mother, Anna, had roots that traced back to the *Mayflower* and had been one of Wesleyan University's last female graduates before the school stopped accepting women in 1902. What the Beebes lacked in money, they made up for in social standing and academic achievement, but Bob was a black sheep whom Joseph had yanked from The Hill and placed in a New York military academy to be toughened up.

After the war, following hospitalization for his fragile temperament, Bob's prospects appeared slim, and he struggled to find work. Once Candace was born, he and Mildred had no choice but to live with the Rosenbergs. For four years, the couple raised their daughter behind the candy store with the help of Mildred's parents, and under Rose's thumb.

By all accounts, while Grandma Rose adored Candace, she was critical and exacting, with a violent temper; once, when Candace disobeyed, her grandmother yanked her wrist so hard that it broke. Rose's fear of scarcity overshadowed daily life, and Candace was often left sitting alone in a high chair at the back of the store, having been told that she couldn't leave until she'd cleaned her plate. After pumping her with food, Rose would then perform horrific enemas and summon doctors for humiliating daily weigh-ins, prompting an ongoing debate over whether Candace was spoiled or sick; accordingly, she would attribute her perpetual struggles with weight to the Rosenbergs' fixation on food.

A born performer and prodigy, Candace entertained candy store patrons by dancing out front, but privately she thrashed against the obsessive focus of her "four parents." Her every move was questioned, and even mundane childhood accidents were the cause of bitter fights. For instance, when Candace climbed over a tent and fell face-first on a stake, causing a deep wound between her eyebrows, a family battle ensued over which doctor to call and whether to get stitches. Candace would later speculate that her parents had been making love, as it was unusual for her to be unsupervised; that would also explain the heightened blame and recrimination by Rose about "The Scar." Afterward, young Candace felt damaged, as relatives cast reproachful glances rather than praising her as the unscathed *shaina maidel*—in Yiddish, a pretty, well-behaved girl—she'd been before.

According to family, Candace inherited smarts from her grandfather, learning math by counting cash with "Poppy" Rosenberg, then stuffing rolls of bills into cigar boxes for pickup. Over time, the Mafia had strong-armed David into running illegal gambling rackets and, though gangsters seemed to love him, the threat of violence was pervasive in the Rosenberg home. Rose knew what fate awaited if her husband failed to deliver, and the family credits her with engendering fortitude in the face of misfortune.

From Rose, Candace acquired strength, as her grandmother pushed women in the family to be educated and independent, reminding them not to rely on men for financial security. "The family was very women-centric, always about empowering the women," says Candace's cousin Nancy Morris, whose mother, Lillian, Mildred's younger sister, became a model and owned a store. "We were taught women could do anything because we had to. It comes from my grandmother. Rose never got soft."

Bob chafed under Rose's command, however, and came to resent his mother-in-law's relentless criticism. As an act of rebellion, he had an affair. While Candace remembered that at age three she entered her parents' bedroom and found her father in bed with a blonde, her family claims that it was Rose who discovered his cheating. Either way, living with the Rosenberg parents proved untenable in the aftermath.

Bob and Mildred reconciled after a short separation, vowing to "break the umbilical cord" and escape the clutches of Grandma Rose. Mildred became pregnant with a second daughter, Wynne, and the young family moved to Levittown, a development on Long Island subsidized by the Veterans Administration and the Federal Housing Administration as affordable housing for returning World War II veterans.

Bob eventually launched an advertising business and became a graphic designer who worked from his garage, but he was always more of an artist than a businessperson, and he balked if clients made requests that rankled his creative sensibilities. Tension brewed when Mildred, who did his billing, forced her husband to make concessions, reminding him that they had kids to feed. The couple often needed their relatives' help to pay the mortgage, and they lacked medical insurance and routine healthcare. All five family members shared a single bathroom. "Candy said that when she got married, she bought her own tweezer and realized they cost nothing," says her youngest sister, Deane Beebe Fitzgerald. "We were always struggling to make ends meet."

In middle age, Bob would dye his thick, Salvador Dalí mustache or comb over his thinning hair to interview for art director positions at advertising agencies. By then, he was rejected for being overqualified and, with no other options, eventually worked as a security guard to provide for the family. To Mildred, this didn't seem fair. Her husband was a polymath and savant whose talent went unrecognized and unrewarded while less impressive friends and neighbors prospered. The couple wrangled privately with disappointment, and the specter of Bob's failed potential hung over the home.

When Candace and her sisters needed clothes, especially for visits to Grandma Rose, their aunt Lillian Glasser stepped in to help. She'd settled less than a mile away after marrying a wealthy accountant who furnished an elevated lifestyle. While the Beebes kept to themselves, Lillian and her husband, Henry, were active members of their temple who socialized with other couples every weekend. Still, Mildred and Lillian remained close, beginning every morning with a phone call to check in, and their children traveled freely between the houses. Though the Beebe girls never received formal religious education or training, they were raised culturally Jewish and celebrated Jewish holidays with the Glassers. If Mildred's children had been male, she would have insisted on bar mitzvahs, but as it was, the Beebes lacked the funds required to join the prominent temple the Glassers attended.

Relatives didn't judge Mildred for observing Christian holidays with Bob as well; after all, she called Christmas "X-mas" to excise the presence of Christ. Plus, the Beebe girls admitted to feeling out of step with their father's WASP kin. When Mildred brought her daughters to visit Bob's family in Connecticut, she wore heels and makeup while her in-laws remained understated and unadorned. Whereas the Rosenberg branch was "huggy-kissy," the Beebes were reserved. Their uncle Bill Beebe gave each child one slice of roast beef with a potato, and they knew never to ask for more, but the Rosenbergs were always pushing food: "Eat, eat, eat! More, more!"

As Candace and her sisters grew older and increasingly self-sufficient, Mildred eased the family's financial burden by returning to work. For years she'd seen professional women gathered at train stations for their daily commute to Manhattan, yet never felt it was possible herself. Given Bob's erratic nature, Mildred lent stability at home and her girls' welfare came first. However, once Candace and her sisters were launched, Mildred came to love her autonomy. She began hosting focus groups to test products on housewives for a market research firm, and then worked in a local library.

Later, Mildred took a full-time job as a clerk typist in Long Island's family and criminal courts, which afforded health benefits for the family, as well as a sense of identity outside her home. She enjoyed dressing up, getting briefed on cases, and admiring the handsome court officers. "My mother said if she'd started working full-time sooner, it would have been a lot easier for us," Deane says. Having seen their mother struggle, the Beebe girls were destined to work.

Notwithstanding their economic hardship, Mildred and Bob loved each other deeply and knew how to make life fun. Bob experimented in the kitchen and, at a time when the most exotic food most families ate was pot roast, he grew an organic garden and would drive to culturally diverse neighborhoods throughout New York in search of unusual ingredients. He'd buy wonton skins to make his own dumplings, or uncommon cuts of meat to prepare on the grill. The couple was open to different cultures, and when Candace worked at the World's Fair and brought home eclectic, international friends, Bob prepared a meal from each visitor's home country.

Though Bob was also an accomplished painter and sculptor, he loved nothing more than music. He played the guitar, piano, and trombone, and even organized a jazz band composed of local high school students who would perform for the neighborhood on a makeshift stage in the Beebes' backyard. "Bob could write a score for a sixteen-piece jazz band on a napkin in the subway," says Steve Bitel, who was two years older than Candace and went to a rival high school. Bitel was hitchhiking one evening and carrying his trombone case when Bob picked him up. When Bob realized that Bitel's music teacher was an army friend, he recruited Bitel to his band.

"Bob was a genius, but he was a wacko too," Bitel continues. "I heard from his army buddy that he would sit on a chair in front of the army chapel stark naked singing 'Onward Christian Soldiers' and playing the cello. He would be three sheets to the wind and have a due date for the next arrangement for the band and he'd be up all night turning it out."

Bob and Mildred were known for being nonconformist. His opium pipes hung over the family's front door, which he'd sometimes answer naked, not knowing who was on the other side. And every Halloween the family dressed in outrageous costumes; one year, Bob posed as a creepy abortionist with Mildred as his patient. Later, when Candace's son Evan surprised Bob by snapping a photo of him sitting on a boat toilet, Bob chose that image for the family's holiday card. The couple was unabashedly themselves, no matter who was watching.

"They were unique and weird and mostly good-hearted, but whoa—what a pair!" says Candace's school friend Nancy Marriott. "I can't remember a time at Candace's house where there wasn't yelling.

Bob was almost abusive at times and out of control, but not in a violent or threatening way. They were just loud." Bob would curse or bloviate on whatever fascinated him, regardless of the reception his diatribes received, and though Mildred was a steadying force, she was also in-your-face. Beaming with a wide-eyed smile, she'd become hyper-present, looking directly into a guest's eyes as though peering into her soul. "She'd say anything off the cuff, whatever was on her mind—not with condemnation or judgment, but she just never held back," Marriott continues. "If Mildred had been my mom, I would have been embarrassed and ashamed. But Candace wasn't. She accepted her."

Despite their volume and intensity, the Beebes' interactions seemed free of animosity. They could fight, chase each other around the house, and even throw things, but then they'd collapse in laughter. Mildred and Bob acknowledged each other's freedom and creativity, and their riotous, no-holds-barred household provided space for each child to express her true nature. This lack of restraint inspired Candace to take risks—or, as Marriott says, "to do something out of the ordinary, and be someone that's never come before."

The Beebe sisters were perceived as follows: Candace was the smart one, Wynne was the pretty one, and Deane was the nice one, a peacemaker who brokered compromises and held the family together. Yet Candace remained the favored child, the apple of her parents' eye. "We were raised that everything was all about Candy," Deane says. "We were all very distinctive and I was so much younger, so it wasn't an issue for me. But Wynne must have had it really hard being in Candy's shadow." While Candace was an animated extrovert, Wynne was sullen and withdrawn, a quiet scowler who would explode in rage and run from the dinner table, at which point Candace would blithely tell guests, "She's just like that." The family bickered constantly, even in front of company, but they also accepted and celebrated each other's differences.

No matter their varying temperaments, Candace adored her sisters and assisted Mildred by walking Deane to school, reading to her, and teaching her to tie her shoes. She also organized inventive games for her younger cousins, and her love of high jinks was apparent from an early age. "You know the scenes from *The Cat in the Hat* when the parents go out? That's what it was like," says cousin Nancy Morris. "Our parents would leave, and bedlam would start. As a kid, it was always something to look forward to."

Candace would lead whipped cream fights, pretend to flush her cousin David down the toilet, or build ice slides on her driveway in winter. One Thanksgiving she placed pots and pans like helmets on her cousins' heads, then steered them outside to throw candy at the house, convincing Grandma Rose that thieves were at the door. On another occasion, when the cousins were visiting their grandparents in Atlantic City, Grandma Rose left freshly baked Passover cookies in a container on the dining room table and forbade the children to touch them. In protest, Candace led her army in trench-crawling past the kitchen to snatch the goodies and then dashing back to a bedroom to devour them. The cousins began throwing pillows in celebration and accidentally bombarded Rose when she walked in, prompting harsh and immediate punishment. "It was always funny," Morris continues. "We would laugh until we cried."

Through her teen years, Candace remained a wild child and joyful provocateur. As a gag, she'd stuff a pillow under her shirt to pretend that she was pregnant, then stroll the Atlantic City boardwalk with her boyfriend as passers-by stared aghast. Having inherited Bob's love of music, if not his proficiency, Candace played the cello in her high school orchestra and flagrantly sat in the front row with her skirt hitched up, the instrument between her legs. Later, upon finding a string quartet at a friend's wedding, she pushed aside the cellist, grabbed his instrument, and again spread her legs, not caring who saw up her dress. And in tenth grade, when Candace learned that the Beatles were playing at Carnegie Hall, she ditched school to sneak backstage into the band's dressing room, where she rifled through their garbage and returned with Ringo's drumsticks, a handful of cigarette butts, and a telegram wishing the Fab Four well on their show.

While Candace was her family's zany ringleader, she could also be manipulative, using her sisters or younger cousins to get what she wanted—and often what she wanted was boys. She'd offer to take her younger sister Deane and a friend to Jones Beach for a day, but instead of watching the girls, Candace would meet her boyfriend for a make-out session in the dunes. A separate time Candace used babysitting as a ploy to visit a boyfriend on Manhattan's Upper West Side. The young man gave Deane and her friend money to buy candy and sent them off to Riverside Park for the day, while he and Candace amused themselves in his apartment. By the time Candace returned home late that night, Mildred and Bob were livid. "Candy loved men," Deane says. "She did what she wanted to do, pretty much always."

Candace's sexuality was core to her being, and she was never afraid to express it. She posed as a nude model for a college art class on figure drawing and delighted in playing strip ghost, a word game akin to strip poker, in which the loser of each round forfeits an article of clothing. Nancy Marriott recalls that at age seventeen, the girls made a pact to lose their virginity at the same time and tell each other about it. "We said it should be special," she recounts. "We didn't get slutty until college."

During the summer of 1965, when Candace and Marriott were nineteen, they shared an apartment in Manhattan and worked at the World's Fair, Candace as a Belgian waffle girl and Marriott as a helicopter stewardess, giving tours. "We were boy-crazy with our birth control pills and women's lib," Marriott says. Because the fair drew an international crowd, they'd say, "Tonight I want a Russian! Tomorrow I'm getting a Dane, the next night a Brit!" A cute Dutchman lived one floor below and, scheming to lure him to their apartment, Candace showed up at his door wearing only sexy lingerie. That same summer, the young women also danced topless in *Relativity*, a short film by Marriott's middle-aged neighbor Ed Emshwiller, an artist and filmmaker.

Mildred and Bob excused their eldest daughter's antics because she was an academic superstar. Candace had applied and been admitted to Smith, Vassar, and the University of Michigan but had chosen Wheaton College in Massachusetts for its full scholarship. After a few months on campus, however, she'd found herself miserable and isolated as she struggled to make friends with the conservative young women in her classes. Candace had been raised in the loving embrace of an extended family who applauded her quirks, and for the first time she felt judged and desperately alone. Following a period of mania during which she subsisted on a diet of peach pie, she was sent home with her parents, who committed her to a local hospital, where she was depressed for several months and prescribed a blend of electroshock therapy and the thyroid-stimulating hormone thyroxine, which proved useless.

The Beebes were distraught over their daughter's "nervous breakdown" and battled over their inability to afford treatment. Yet they expected her to stabilize and rematriculate at another top school, and thus were further alarmed by her slapdash romance with Agu Pert. While contemplating her future, Candace had enrolled at Hofstra University because it was close to her family's home. She met Agu in the fall of 1965 when she began assisting in the lab where he worked as a graduate student, applying scientific principles to the study of human behavior to earn his master's degree in experimental psychology, a precursor to neuroscience.

When Agu first saw Candace among the cages of his professor's exotic animals—kinkajous, coatimundis, Gila monsters, pythons, king vultures, and a gibbon—she seemed a rare creature herself. He was immediately attracted to this striking young woman with long, tan legs, wearing shorts. He asked Candace for a cigarette one afternoon and quickly discovered that, far from being a mere "shiny thing," she vibrated with a free spirit and burning intellect. "Candace was open and gregarious, unbelievably vital, full of energy and life. She had no inhibitory filters. What you saw was what you got, which is sometimes refreshing and sometimes tiring," says Agu, who is by nature quiet and polite, straitlaced and understated—in many ways the opposite of Candace, yet equally ardent.

Immediately, Agu was overcome by the exhilaration of new love, the feeling that he'd connected and resonated so completely as to be irrevocably consumed. It was an unforgettable high, he says, with memories that linger forever. From their first beer at Ryan's Pub just off campus, Candace and Agu were inseparable, spending every minute together, discussing their future's endless possibilities. Candace told Agu about her breakdown almost immediately and confided that, while she'd stopped taking medication, she felt confident in her full recovery. At the time, Agu was unconcerned about Candace's mental health; if anything, her weakness activated his self-confessed "white knight syndrome," a masculine urge to rescue and protect, and her madcap nature made each day feel like an adventure.

"We could not get enough of being together," Agu recounts. "We talked about everything. It was a very passionate relationship." So passionate that, two months later, on November 7, when the couple was caught during a blackout in Room 007 in Phillips Hall, they made love on the laboratory floor. Weeks later, when Candace felt nauseous at a movie theater during *Thunderball*, she was savvy enough not to blame

James Bond or the meal she and Agu had shared before a roaring fire-place at 17 Barrow Street, a romantic restaurant in Greenwich Village. While the couple suspected it was morning sickness, they avoided the truth until an obstetrician confirmed that they had, indeed, conceived a child. "We were both kind of irresponsible, not very orthodox," Agu reflects. He was twenty-six and Candace a mere nineteen.

Agu and Candace never considered getting an abortion because they were already secretly engaged. In December he'd given her a Linde sapphire ring with a few small diamonds that he'd purchased on a payment plan for $125, and, like Mildred and Bob before them, they'd conspired to elope. On March 18, 1966, the couple told their parents that they were going to a seminar at a shark lab in Sandy Hook, New Jersey, then drove with the top down in his Oldsmobile convert-ible to the Nassau County courthouse. Agu's taciturn professor, whom he'd invited to bear witness, read the *New York Times* while Candace and Agu deliberated with a judge who initially refused to marry them because their parents were absent. Ironically, when Agu had arrived in a suit to pick up Candace at her family home, Mildred had laughed, remarking that the couple looked like they were about to get hitched. Little did she know.

After the ceremony, Agu had $100 to spend on a pizza reception at the bowling alley next door. The newlyweds then hopped into Agu's car, put the top down, turned the radio up, and drove to the Bronx Zoo, where, giddy with excitement and hope, they held hands and wandered among the animals. On their return to Long Island, they stopped at a restaurant and nightclub on Jericho Turnpike in Mineola that Agu envisioned as a bastion for the elite but which turned out to be a Mafia hangout where a comedian performed jokes in Italian. Following a rich meal with the Cosa Nostra, the couple spent the next two days at a Syosset motel, leaving bed only to eat.

Vowing to keep their shotgun wedding a secret, they removed their rings and stuck them in the trunk of Agu's car before retreating to their respective homes. Less than two weeks later, however, Mildred's friend saw the couple's marriage posted in *Newsday*'s court record and phoned her with the news. Mildred, in turn, called Agu's mother, Elsa, who flew into a rage.

To Elsa, a conservative immigrant who'd escaped Estonia during World War II on the strength of her father's German citizenship, her son marrying a Jew felt like an affront. When Agu was a baby, she'd had only a day to decide whether to leave her family to flee with retreating German troops, and she'd relied on the kindness of German strangers when she and her son landed in a foreign town in the southwestern federal state of Baden-Württemberg. Elsa had worked in a factory making parts for military equipment by day and endured British bombs at night. Sometimes she and Agu would wander into fields surrounding their village and stare at a sky ablaze in orange as the nearby city of Pforzheim was razed.

When World War II ended, millions of displaced people were shuttled into camps around Europe as governments debated where they would live. Those who'd escaped Communist-occupied countries would be shot or sent to Siberia if they dared return, so Elsa and Agu were fortunate to land in a camp specifically for Estonians located in a sector of Germany administratively controlled by Americans. For four years, they waited to hear whether they would be sent to the United States, Canada, Australia, or Sweden. Finally, in 1949, under the terms of the Displaced Persons Act, they were sponsored by an Estonian family and joined eleven thousand refugees from their homeland admitted into the United States between 1948 and 1952.

Agu and his mother lived for a few months in Harlem on West 124th Street before Elsa found a job as a live-in domestic for a prominent

Spanish diplomat in tony Locust Valley, on Long Island. "It didn't work out because my mother didn't put up with shit," Agu says. "At that point, she'd been through quite a lot. She was one of the most amazing people, an unbelievably strong person to have gone through what she did." Before long, Elsa found work as a maid and cook at a paper baron's estate in Old Westbury, and her wealthy patrons helped procure a green card for Elsa's former Estonian lover, Arthur Orav, with whom she'd reunited when he arrived illegally in the United States. When Agu's mother and stepfather married, the family moved to Baldwin, where Arthur joined an Estonian construction crew. Because communication was cut while the Iron Curtain was in place, Agu learned only in his thirties that his birth father, August Pert, was still alive.

While the Beebes were fervently antiwar, particularly given American incursions in Vietnam, Agu had channeled his gratitude for the sanctuary granted to his family by enlisting in his college's undergraduate ROTC program. Intending to become both "an officer and a gentleman," he'd completed his college language requirement in Russian and dreamed of joining the army's Special Forces with mysterious deployments in the Baltic states. At the time, Agu even deemed Simon and Garfunkel subversive and had voted for Barry Goldwater, the Republican senator from Arizona, in the 1964 presidential election. He also still needed to satisfy his ROTC military requirement, and given Bob's torturous tour in World War II, the Beebes dreaded the effects of a deployment.

Considering Agu's heritage, Aryan appearance, and fervent patriotism, Mildred and Lillian were overwrought for months, imagining a Nazi had just married into their family. "In my family, there weren't a lot of closed-door conversations. It was all out there. You heard everything over the dinner table—except this," Deane says. "It was earth-shattering." However, since the Beebes had caused a scandal with their own pairing, Candace's mother eventually saw past Agu's fair complexion and shy demeanor, but only after confirming that Agu and Elsa had escaped both Communists and Nazis and were not fans of either.

Still, Mildred's daughters were her trophies and her eldest was a rising star, so the Beebes worried that Candace's pregnancy would derail her education and job prospects. Fearing that Candace would suffer a fate worse than Bob's if she got off track, Mildred insisted that she not squander her natural gifts. "When she got pregnant, my mother was like, 'Where's your career? What's going to become of you?'" Deane says. Once Evan was born, however, he took center stage and was showered with affection; and when, two days after his birth on August 8, 1966, the *New York Times* published an article with the headline "Births Up 9 Months After the Blackout," the family learned that he was one of many children conceived that November night.

Just as her family grew comfortable with Agu, Candace scandalized them again by deciding to drop out of college to follow her husband to Pennsylvania. As an ROTC reserve officer, Agu was expected to serve in the Vietnam War, but reports from the front were horrifying and Agu shuddered at leaving his new wife and baby. To avoid being drafted, he'd decided to pursue his doctorate, choosing Bryn Mawr College for its prestigious psychology department and healthy stipend for a PhD candidate.

The couple packed everything they owned into a U-Haul and moved to a one-bedroom, ground-floor apartment within walking distance of the suburban campus. After subtracting the $85-per-month rent, they had $115 per month to live on, so Candace spent her days experimenting with recipes from *The Joy of Cooking* and caring for Evan, following advice from Dr. Benjamin Spock's famous child-rearing book.

Candace and Agu agreed that this relocation wouldn't mark the end of her education, but she had no clear plans to rematriculate and soon grew restless from a lack of intellectual stimulation. She considered taking night classes at Temple University in Philadelphia, but with money tight she soon sought work, first selling cosmetics three nights per week at Wanamaker's department store in the King of Prussia mall, and then waiting tables at the Haverford Hot Shoppe, where she had the good fortune to serve a Bryn Mawr dean of admissions. After delivering the dean's food, Candace mentioned that her husband was a graduate student and that she wished to resume her studies. Upon learning of her standout grades and SAT scores, the dean invited her to interview the following day.

"Candace was unbelievably sociable and extroverted, and she talked her way into Bryn Mawr," Agu recalls with a smile. "She could talk her way into anything." She was accepted at the end of August and offered a break on tuition but, with classes starting just a week later, the couple still scrambled for a bank loan to cover Bryn Mawr's $1,500 bill. That fall, Candace commenced a heavy course load that included advanced calculus, chemistry, biology, and physics, which proved to be the first time she'd been challenged academically. Bryn Mawr, Agu says, was exactly where she belonged.

At Wheaton and Hofstra, Candace had declared a major in English with hopes of becoming a magazine editor. Yet she'd become disgruntled after receiving a C-minus on a paper titled "The Greek Mind." Candace thought it a masterpiece, but when her professor disagreed, she grew frustrated by the subjective nature of written work. There was no black or white, no right or wrong, and despite her best efforts, the professor couldn't see her case. In contrast, Agu's world of science felt clear and linear. During the couple's nightly discussions, Candace had developed a fascination with the inner workings of the brain and had found herself reading Agu's textbooks for fun. She'd loved the biology class she'd taken at Hofstra, so she chose this concentration at Bryn Mawr.

Though she excelled in her classes, Candace was discouraged from pursuing science, particularly by female professors. As she recounts in *Molecules of Emotion*, the few women who survived in this arena did so by donning the armor of men, assuming a persona Candace calls "the science nun." These severe scholars sported an all-black uniform, pulled their hair tightly into buns, and banished all evidence of frivolity or femininity to prove they were just as robust as male peers. Upon learning that Candace was already a married mother at age twenty, they clucked that she'd never last in their competitive world. To prove naysayers wrong, Candace survived on little rest, often sleeping only from 6 a.m. to noon, which was the only time available after classes, labs, homework, dinners with Agu, and caring for Evan.

Candace and Agu fancied themselves a modern couple, a scientific team who aimed to make strides together. Atypically for men of his generation, Agu encouraged his wife to achieve, in part because he spent two years as a "warden" or dorm parent at Bryn Mawr, developing sympathy for the talented young women in his care. Generally, wardens were either young faculty or advanced graduate students, and Agu and Candace had been invited for their capacity to provide a trusted, familial environment. The position came with a stipend that doubled Agu's research assistantship and provided a free place to live, along with free phone usage and meals with students while school was in session. Though Candace was an undergraduate herself, she managed to gain the respect of her peers because her life experiences and responsibilities were sufficiently weighty. She became a confidant to anyone who asked for her advice, and fellow students loved hearing Evan sing Woody Guthrie's "This Land Is Your Land" while strumming his toy guitar in the dorm's common room at night.

While Agu found his initial interactions with his new charges awkward and intimidating as they approached him with distinctly female troubles, he was shaped by these students, as most had progressive ideas that challenged his own political leanings. Influenced by Candace and her peers, Agu voted for Hubert Humphrey for president in 1968 and participated in anti–Vietnam War marches and protests in Bryn Mawr and at Rittenhouse Square in Philadelphia, without regard for the consequences he'd face as an army officer with a deferral. A minority in the company of gifted women, Agu also grew to understand the female perspective. "Living with fifty young, extremely bright ladies set the foundation for my later transformation into an ardent feminist," he says.

Rather than feeling threatened by his wife, Agu marveled at her ability to shift from right to left brain. Candace brought art into science, and while Agu believed "she could do anything," in those days "anything" for women meant aspiring to teach. God forbid anyone thought of women in a lab. Yet Bryn Mawr had instilled in Candace a love of scientific research, and after she earned her diploma cum laude, she aspired to do graduate work in biology at either Johns Hopkins or the University of Delaware, to which she could commute from Agu's post at Edgewood Arsenal, forty minutes north of Baltimore, where he would fulfill his military requirement by evaluating the long-term effects of nerve gas poisoning and searching for antidotes. Candace's Hopkins application was rejected, however, after an interviewer learned that she had a young child and a husband who, at a moment's notice, might be summoned to serve in Vietnam. With her duties as wife and mother, he averred, she couldn't possibly commit to biomedicine.

Though Candace seemed destined for Delaware, her life seldom went according to plan, and fortuitous events soon changed her fate. When she and Agu attended the annual Federation of American Societies for Experimental Biology conference in Atlantic City, Candace caught wind of a young prodigy, Dr. Solomon Snyder. Coincidentally,

Snyder's name came up again after she'd returned to Bryn Mawr, when the couple attended a psychology department lecture. Their speaker that evening was Dr. Joe Brady, a colorful psychologist who, as a U.S. Army captain, had founded the department of experimental psychology at Walter Reed Army Medical Center and was now a professor of behavioral biology, conducting studies on the physiological effects of stress in monkeys at the Johns Hopkins medical school. At a party that followed, someone began playing an old 78 rpm record of Peabody dance music and Brady sought a partner. Though Candace had never danced the Peabody, she had a natural sense of rhythm and commanded the floor until she and Brady collapsed in a sweaty heap.

In conversation afterward, when Candace confided her wish to study the brain, Brady lit up; he knew just the guy she had to meet, he said, and offered to hand-deliver her résumé. Upon reading Candace's fawning cover letter expressing her "fondest dreams and desires," Sol Snyder called with an offer uncannily akin to the Bryn Mawr dean's—a position in his lab as a doctoral candidate, along with a research assistantship that provided a stipend and waived all tuition.

"You're accepted," Snyder said. "Now apply."

CHAPTER THREE

THE PRINCE

THE MORNING AFTER CANDACE'S OPIATE RECEPTOR DISCOVERY, WHEN SNYDER returned from his conference, his reluctance dissolved the moment she slapped the data on his desk. For a beat, he stared silently at her numbers, and then sprang from his chair. "Fuck! Fuck! Fuck!" he cried, pacing around the office, brewing plans. Yes, Candace had shown stereospecific binding, he said, but that alone was not enough to declare victory. Before announcing publicly that they'd found the opiate receptor, they needed to perform additional experiments to systematically confirm. And they'd better hurry, lest they be scooped by rivals.

Night and day, Candace began working toward her goal, stretching her resources and goading underlings. Adele Snowman, the gifted technician assigned to assist, often joined Candace in the lab at 5 a.m. They worked twelve-hour days and on weekends, and Candace frequently called her at 10 p.m. with some new insight. "She would always come up with something unusual and I'd scratch my head and think, 'I don't know about this.' But we had the luxury to try new things because it was uncharted territory," Snowman recalls. "I've never worked in any lab that's been as exciting. I didn't mind working my butt off. I grew very attached to this project as well. It became my child."

First Candace and Adele surveyed more than fifty opiate drugs to see whether their effect on binding sites would correspond with their relative potencies, which they did. As receptor theory suggested, the more potent the drug, the more aggressively it competed with an antagonist to lodge inside receptors. They also tested non-opiate substances such as serotonin, caffeine, and histamine, none of which attached to these sites, illustrating that the receptors they'd found were highly selective. Next, after initially using intestinal strips, they performed assays on brain tissue and were thrilled to discover opiate receptors distributed throughout the brain's regions in varying densities; areas such as the corpus striatum and limbic system were rich in opiate receptors, which would lend insight into how opiates manipulate pain perception or mood, and why the opiate receptor exists in the first place.

Once Snyder deemed Candace's evidence incontrovertible, it was time to write. In big-league science, it's not enough to make a discovery; a scientist must plant her flag by announcing findings in a prestigious scientific journal, as publication and subsequent citations of one's work by others are vital to cementing a career. Candace and Snyder's paper, "Opiate Receptor: Demonstration in Nervous Tissue," appeared in *Science*, the most widely read scientific journal in America, just five months later, on March 9, 1973. Candace was listed first, as the subordinate responsible for the majority of work, and Snyder was named second as the senior author who'd provided oversight and funding.

The response was overwhelming. Johns Hopkins, in coordination with the nearby National Institute of Mental Health, issued a press release heralding a "major breakthrough that could lead to a better treatment for narcotics addiction," and hosted a national press conference the same day in Baltimore. Candace and Snyder were mobbed by network and local TV and print reporters firing questions both scientific and political. The *New York Times*, *Washington Post*, and *Newsweek* all featured stories, as did the Associated Press and United Press International. Though some venues went so far as to trumpet a "magic bullet" for drug dependence, Candace was quoted as saying, "What we have is not a cure for heroin addiction, but something that may lead us to a faster cure than we had hoped."

Immediately, factions vied to take credit for Candace and Snyder's work. Despite its war on drugs, the Nixon administration had been trying to curtail the budget of the National Institutes of Health, the nation's federally funded medical research agency, claiming that basic medical research seldom delivers results with practical applications. To fend off politicians' encroachment, William "Biff" Bunney, who was directing drug abuse research at the NIH, saw an opening to claim a win for science and safeguard his endowment. The Nixon administration, in turn, was eager to assert that the opiate receptor discovery was the direct result of its efforts to end addiction.

The Republican Party also appealed to Big Pharma by touting efficiencies that would speed the development of new drugs, as Candace's technique in test tubes was faster and cheaper than methods used by drug companies at the time. Until now, pharmaceutical firms had measured the effects of psychoactive drugs exclusively on live animals; even a simple assay required fifty to a hundred rats that cost $5 apiece and required higher doses of each drug, not to mention weeks of a chemist's valuable time. In contrast, using Candace's receptor-binding technique, skilled technicians like Adele Snowman could screen for five thousand separate drugs using the brain of a single rat.

Test tube screening also allowed companies to create dozens of molecular variants to refine a drug's potency and selectivity; finding the lowest possible dose at which a drug proved therapeutic would help reduce side effects when administered in humans. "This technique was so quick, easy, and reproducible," Snowman says. "I could do two thousand samples and get so much data in one day with her method. It was an incredible time, and it changed the dynamics of our research lab."

Almost overnight, Sol Snyder emerged as a power broker, presiding over a lab that flourished, Candace said, "like Florence in the Renaissance." Zealous students clamored for admission, and grants were funded with barely a second look. With increased resources, Snyder was no longer content to focus solely on addiction; instead, he would leverage Candace's "receptor technology" to expand his purview to the mind, the central nervous system, and the entire body. After all, receptors had evolved not for exogenous drugs but for our body's internal chemicals like hormones and neurotransmitters. And if opiates had receptors, then other drugs did too. Snyder intended to find them.

The procedure Candace had spent months tweaking and honing was employed universally by her peers in Snyder's lab to detect, in quick succession, receptors for the neurotransmitter glycine, which affects motor neurons in the spinal cord and may impact stroke victims; acetylcholine, which has implications for Alzheimer's disease; norepinephrine, which affects memory, focus, and blood pressure; dopamine, which governs motivation and reward-seeking; serotonin, which regulates emotional behavior; and the GABA receptor of the central nervous system. One after another, Candace's colleagues found them all.

Still, Snyder made sure to assign Candace the projects poised to yield the biggest breakthroughs. She had at her disposal copious resources generally reserved for faculty members and continued to thrive under Snyder's tutelage, studying the brains of rat fetuses to reveal that opiate receptors develop before birth, thereby proving that mammals may become addicted in the womb. Moreover, following their initial press conference, Snyder had received untold invitations to speak at conferences and universities all over the world. But instead of traveling the globe himself, he'd emboldened Candace, a lowly graduate student, to assume the spotlight within the "Opiate Club," as the group of long-standing researchers in this field was called.

"It was amazing to see her develop as a world-class scientist. It was fun that she was recognized and admired most everywhere. Essentially, she was the founder of neural receptor research," Agu says, emphasizing that when pharmaceutical companies want to screen a drug for psychoactive properties today, they still use the same receptor binding techniques that Candace pioneered. "It was a heady time and it got better. We were able to go to all these cool conventions in Mexico, Scotland, Italy. You felt like you'd really made it and were top of the world at these clubs."

Following completion of her graduate work in 1974, Candace scripted a glowing tribute to Snyder in her doctoral dissertation, expressing gratitude for the privilege of working with him, praising his "kindness, consideration, and generosity," and calling him "a dedicated teacher with an uncanny talent for defining the critical scientific question, designing the 'right' experiment, disregarding the irrelevant or misleading result, and drawing the essential conclusion." Instead of moving to a separate laboratory for her postdoctoral work, as is customary, she remained at Hopkins to continue her opiate research alongside her mentor and his colleagues.

From Mike Kuhar, a junior professor and expert in neuroanatomy who occupied the lab next to Snyder's, Candace learned a technique called autoradiography, in which X-ray film is used to picture molecules or fragments of molecules with radioactive tracers. A radioactive opiate is injected into an animal's brain, and then a thin slice of brain is exposed to X-ray film. Radioactive molecules produce silver grains on the film, generating a map of the exact locations of opiate receptors in various sections of the brain. Using this method, Candace found an abundance of opiate receptors in the limbic system, with particularly dense clusters in the amygdala. Because the limbic system controls emotions, she and Snyder extrapolated that these receptors were linked to opiates' effect on mood.

After uncovering concentrations of opiate receptors in the peri-aqueductal gray (PAG) in the midbrain and in the medial thalamus, regions known to regulate pain perception, they reasoned that opiate drugs target these areas for pain relief. What's more, after determining that the substantia gelatinosa, which runs along the backside of the spinal cord, is also rich in opiate receptors, Candace and Snyder proved that opiates mitigate pain in the central nervous system as well as in the brain. They even discerned why opiates cause euphoria, slow breathing, and constrict the pupils of the eye.

In just a few years, Candace and Snyder had opened the door to a whole new field of research, understanding with precision the inner workings of the brain. This was "hot science" at its best, and some of the world's most prominent researchers began to flood this cutting-edge arena. With competition suddenly fierce, Snyder was determined to defend his turf. Thus, as Candace prepared to leave Hopkins, she noted friction with her boss. The rub had begun earlier, when Snyder had shared Candace's technique with her lab mates, enabling them to capitalize on it as well. The discovery of each new receptor had diverted Snyder's attention and ignited Candace's jealousy. This project was her obsession, a baby she had birthed and wanted to raise herself, not share with her peers. Why should they reap the spoils of her labor?

Distributing credit around his lab made Snyder not only a sensible manager but also a shrewd politician. Prior to Candace's discovery, the lab had no particular acclaim, and now Snyder was known the world over. For a lab chief, this outcome is ideal, as leaders strive to hire subordinates whose work will bolster their credentials. "When I was recruiting graduate students to my lab, [a mentor] said to me, 'Hire this guy because he'll make you famous,'" Agu recalls. "That's how it was done." Candace had made Snyder famous, and many colleagues whispered that without her he would be a well-respected neuroscientist but would never have become a titan. One way to ensure that recognition remained with Snyder, rather than traveling with Candace, was to shift the spotlight away from his star pupil.

In the years that followed, Snyder would receive a bevy of prestigious awards, including the John Gaddum Memorial Award from the British Pharmacological Society, the Daniel H. Efron Research Award from the American College of Neuropsychopharmacology, and the Van Giesen Award from Columbia University. He was appointed Cambridge University's Sir Henry Dale Centennial Lecturer and the University of Wisconsin's Rennebohm Lecturer. In 1977, he'd be appointed Distinguished Service Professor at Hopkins; in 1978, he'd become president of the Society for Neuroscience; and by 1980, Snyder would take the helm of Hopkins's Department of Neuroscience, the university's first new science department in twenty years.

Candace was thrilled to have propelled her mentor's rise and strove to make him proud, like Snyder had for Julius Axelrod, and Axelrod had for Steve Brodie. Yet what appeared to be a "classic mentor-disciple, father-child transition" escalated on her final day at Hopkins when, as Candace was saying goodbye, Snyder asked her to abandon any further work related to the opiate receptor.

Of course, she felt devastated by this unfair request, and she wondered whether she had ignited Snyder's jealousy with her frequent speaking engagements and media appearances. Now that Candace wouldn't be under Snyder's thumb, did he perceive her ambition as a threat? As she recounts in *Molecules of Emotion*, in that instant she remembered an episode a few months prior when Snyder had inquired if she'd ever read *The Prince* by Machiavelli. "You really should read the chapter about killing the king," he told her. "If one is going to kill the king, then one should never wound him, but finish the job and be done with it."

Three years would pass before Candace absorbed the weight of her mentor's words. By then, she was in full swing at the NIMH. Candace had hidden her second pregnancy while applying for ten positions and had received offers from the University of Florida at Gainesville, the University of Chicago, and the NIMH. She'd joined the NIMH in September 1975 as a staff fellow in the section on biochemistry and pharmacology of the Biological Psychiatry Branch because Agu had also received an offer in the exceptional, tenure-track intramural program there. The couple would share a laboratory in Bethesda.

Once ensconced in her lab in the NIMH's Building 10, Candace found that her high-profile work attracted top collaborators and students. Bucking Snyder's request, she continued the receptor research she'd begun at Hopkins and was instrumental in characterizing peptides, or short strings of amino acids (typically between two and fifty) that form the building blocks of proteins. Candace and her team isolated neuropeptides such as neurotensin, which is found in both the central nervous system and the gut; bombesin, which plays a role in smooth muscle contraction, cell growth, and endocrine responses; and vasoactive intestinal peptide, which is synthesized by immune cells.

"It was a revolution in neurobiology. It opened the floodgates," says Miles Herkenham, a neuroanatomist with whom Candace also conceived of an autoradiographic technique to view receptors alongside neural pathways. "Candace was scientifically very productive, with an active, busy lab that produced good progeny and attracted good people who recognized that this was a research opportunity gold mine."

Meanwhile, Candace knew that Snyder's efforts were focused on finding the opiate receptor's reason for being—the body's natural pain-killer. "We can assume that nature did not put opiate receptors in the brain solely to interact with narcotics," Snyder had told *Newsweek*, and he and Candace had speculated about a morphine-like ligand that inter-acts with the opiate receptor to alleviate pain. But it had yet to be found in the body. Seasoned "Opiate Club" researchers, such as Hans Koster-litz, a pharmacologist who had fled Hitler's Germany, and his associ-ate John Hughes at the University of Aberdeen in Scotland, had long been searching for the body's natural morphine when Snyder began his quest. After learning that they'd shown early results in pig brains, Sny-der's gung-ho spirit was piqued, and he ramped up efforts in his lab.

Regardless, the Aberdeen team bested Snyder, publishing an article in the British journal *Nature* in December 1975 declaring that they'd identified the chemical structure for a ligand they called enkephalin, from a Greek term meaning "in the head." Later, the American nomen-clature "endorphin" (short for endogenous morphine) would take hold, but for now this triumph was savored by the Brits. Snyder yielded to sportsmanship, acknowledging his peers' victory with a magnum of Harrod's finest Cognac—and, some suspect, greasing the wheels for a gentlemen's agreement that would rattle the scientific establishment.

At the time, Candace was desperate to believe the best about her mentor; he'd been a father figure, after all, and she couldn't fathom that he'd block her ascent. So she was blindsided when, in March 1977, Snyder published an article in *Scientific American,* "Opiate Receptors and Internal Opiates," which listed him as sole author and made no mention of Candace's work. She knew that this popular publication had a wide circulation and paid hefty fees of $5,000 to $10,000 per article, and she felt stung to be denied credit and money Snyder knew would aid her growing family.

Then, in the spring of 1978, John Hughes, the more junior of the Aberdeen duo, stopped by Candace's home to inform, or possibly warn, her that he and his boss Kosterlitz, along with Snyder, were to receive the Lasker Award in October for their opiate work. The Lasker is America's highest scientific honor and many of its winners are subsequently awarded the Nobel Prize, so Candace assumed that there had to be some mistake. Given her role in the opiate receptor discovery, which had transformed the field of neuroscience, it simply wasn't possible that she'd be excluded.

Despite Snyder's maneuver in *Scientific American*, Candace naively ignored Hughes's admonition until her mentor called personally to invite her to the Lasker luncheon in New York City—as his guest. This slight was too much to bear; the idea that she would sit clapping in the crowd while Snyder, who had tried to abort her project, was showered with accolades seemed horribly unfair.

Unfair, but not unprecedented, since female scientists were regularly second-guessed, overlooked, and denigrated. Most notably, Francis Crick and John Watson had filched an X-ray diffraction image from the skilled British chemist Rosalind Franklin, enabling them to demonstrate DNA's double helix structure and thereby win the 1962 Nobel Prize. Watson had even chronicled and justified their theft in his book *The Double Helix*. "I woke up one morning and looked in the mirror," Candace writes, "only to find Rosalind Franklin looking back at me. . . . No, I told myself, I couldn't let this happen, to be forgotten and ignored by history, while the boys waltzed away with the prize."

However, when Candace surveyed her colleagues, they advised her to stay silent, maintaining that this was "how the game is played." It is customary for lab chiefs to receive awards for successful experiments they've funded or directed and that underlings perform. And, they argued, John Hughes held a rank senior to Candace's; he was an assistant professor who had been sole author on various papers on enkephalin, while she had been a mere graduate student. Regardless, Candace believed that since she and Hughes appeared in the same first-author position on their respective opiate papers, this rationale didn't hold water.

When Candace appealed directly to Snyder, begging him to reject the award in protest or to give half of his prize money to her alma mater Bryn Mawr, he demurred, chalking up Candace's omission to an error by the Lasker committee and claiming he'd been removed from the process; he sympathized with Candace, he said, but it simply wasn't his fault. However, while Snyder had been technically nominated by the chair of Hopkins's pharmacology department, Candace and Agu say that a colleague with whom she'd studied autoradiography at Hopkins called her to report that he'd seen on Snyder's desk that he'd written his own nomination, or at least the first draft. "Of course, Candace's name was not on it," Agu says. "It was because she was younger and because she was a woman."

Besides, everyone knew Snyder had his eye on the Nobel Prize, and Nobel rules stipulate that only three scientists can win a single award. Snyder's mentor, Julius Axelrod, had even petitioned Candace to help him prepare a Nobel nomination for Snyder, Kosterlitz, and Hughes, vowing that Snyder would help her later. "That's how science recognition works," Axelrod had reasoned. Perhaps for men, Candace thought, but not for women like her and Rosalind Franklin.

Historically, women had no recourse; they simply didn't fight back. But Candace did fight. Ostracized by the mighty male cabal to which she'd aspired, she now sought sisters in arms whose fury matched hers, and who would be sympathetic to her plight or help amplify her voice. Candace penned a fervent letter to the Lasker committee explaining her position, and Agu mailed a copy to Jean Marx, an editor at *Science*, who promptly wrote an editorial, "Lasker Award Stirs Controversy," that triggered other journalists, many of them women, to take up Candace's cause. In February 1979, Joan Arehart-Treichel of *Science News* revealed that no one, not even Snyder, had ever mentioned Candace as a potential Lasker candidate; in fact, the first the Lasker committee had heard of her was when Arehart-Treichel presented them with a copy of Candace and Snyder's paper.

To address speculation that Candace had been a student merely following instructions from her respected boss, many noted her subsequent achievements. For instance, while researching the peptides of enkephalin (endorphins) after their 1977 discovery, Candace discerned that they decompose rapidly in the body. This meant that the body's natural painkiller doesn't last long, so if doctors wanted to produce a long-acting analgesic, they would need to improve upon nature. Once again beating her competition to the punch, Candace found that by substituting a different amino acid (d-alanine instead of l-alanine) in the number two position in the chain of five peptides that forms the body's native morphine, she could slow its degradation to manage pain for prolonged periods.

Though the pharmaceutical giant Burroughs Wellcome was busy configuring hundreds of variations on enkephalin in an effort to manufacture a nonaddictive pain reliever, its scientists had no such *aha* moment. However, because the company had patented its alternative structures, Candace's patent was rejected on the grounds that Burroughs Wellcome had filed first, even if their researchers had missed the import of their findings. Regardless, "Candace's contribution was ingenious," Agu says. "The only reason they figured out what they had was because Candy showed them."

What's more, in May 1979 Eugene Garfield of the Institute for Scientific Information analyzed Candace's ongoing contribution to her field in terms of her papers published and the number of citations

she'd received. Like footnotes or appendices in a book, scientific citations are acknowledgments to authors of preceding papers, a record
of interdependence between the latest research and all relevant prior
work. By mapping citations, Garfield concluded that in the publish-or-
perish realm of academic medicine, "Pert's work at NIMH continues
to be significant to her colleagues" and "she is still a force within the
specialty without the help of her mentor." Garfield also found that the
papers Snyder had coauthored with Candace during her time at Hopkins received more than twice as many citations as papers Snyder had
published with others. This, he deduced, was strong evidence that
Candace deserved formal recognition.

Additionally, in April 1979, at the height of the Lasker controversy,
Dr. Bill Pollin, the director of the National Institute on Drug Abuse
(NIDA), submitted a note to *Science* acknowledging that this was
not the first time Candace had been excluded from an award given to
someone else based on her work. Two years prior, NIDA had bestowed
its Pacesetter Award on Avram Goldstein, John Hughes, Hans Koster-
litz, Eric Simon, Solomon Snyder, and Lars Terenius for their development of concepts and characterization of the structure and function of
enkephalin.

"In retrospect, we feel that it was a significant omission on our
part that Dr. Candace Pert was not included. Her graduate student
role was the issue at the time; subsequent increased awareness of her
major contribution has led us to this revised conclusion," Pollin wrote.
"Selecting recipients for prestigious awards is a complex social process
in which 'scientific merit,' unfortunately, is often only one of many con-
siderations. Sometimes, serious mistakes are made."

Still, while ample evidence pointed to Snyder's duplicity, which
Candace depicts as premeditated, the question of whether there was
cut-and-dried wrongdoing is likely more nuanced, with perspectives

diverging even among her female peers. Credit in science is often hard to assign, as progress is incremental and cumulative, with each minor discovery building upon the next before a game-changing development can occur. Scientific progress never occurs in a vacuum, and every seemingly overnight success is often the product of a decade of hard labor, with senior scientists shepherding each new generation of graduate students or postdocs toward a series of milestones.

To achieve her great leap forward with the opiate receptor, Candace had synthesized the ideas of others. She'd immersed herself in Avram Goldstein's formative text; adopted Pedro Cuatrecasas's rapid filtration system; and spent nights batting around ideas with Agu, who had found in his work at Edgewood Arsenal, where he was implanting cannulas in the brains of rhesus monkeys to determine where drugs act in the brain, that the periaqueductal gray is where pain is perceived. Yet when Candace "skimmed the cream" to nab the final accolade, none of these influential sources got credit. She alone became a star.

Even Agu concedes that Candace's work would have been impossible without Snyder's input. His creativity and intelligence were undeniable, and he'd become entranced with the opiate receptor after reading Avram Goldstein's paper and hearing him speak. Snyder had written the grant, procured funding, and had the connections to promote their discovery. His relationship with Candace was symbiotic, so they should have shared acclaim. "She didn't come up with the idea for the project, but she was the one to implement it," Agu says. "I know Candace took the naloxone without Sol's permission or knowledge because she got it from me. I don't think Sol admits to this day exactly what happened."

Given the atmosphere of cutthroat gamesmanship Snyder cultivated in his lab, some speculate that he'd created a Frankenstein's monster in Candace, stoking her ego until she strove to surpass him.

Though Snyder's workspace was electrifying, it was also competitive to the point of hostility, with power-hungry glory-mongering modeled from the top down. Snyder strategically pitted peers against each other, and his lab was marked by stewing resentments and turf wars erupting almost daily. Trainees were secretive with other trainees, and each year Snyder planned a meeting whose express purpose was collaboration and information-sharing with another lab, yet instructed his protégés beforehand, "Don't say too much!"

Snyder had prepared Candace for the vicious clash for credit endemic to high-stakes science, teaching her to exploit and publicize her findings for maximum impact. This meant marginalizing the contributions of others. In her memoir, Candace admits that she and Sol intentionally excluded any meaningful reference to Avram Goldstein's groundwork in their paper on the opiate receptor, though ethics necessitated a mention. Snyder, however, ascribed it to a need for brevity, as most papers published in *Science* are a mere fifteen hundred words. Either way, their omission rankled Goldstein, enough that he sent Snyder a letter rebuking him for being "ungenerous."

"I have found—and being older than you can offer fatherly-type advice—that it enhances rather than diminishes one's scientific stature to lean over backward in acknowledging precedents and priorities," Goldstein chided. "The work you reported would have seemed just as important and significant had you discussed its relationship to our investigations in a more constructive way."

Colleagues describe Snyder as a consummate political animal, not wired for munificence. While racing against the Aberdeen team to find the chemical structure of endorphins, he and Candace had also led John Hughes "like a lamb to the slaughter," persuading him to undermine himself by sharing key findings prematurely at a conference in Boston. Steeped in her mentor's commands, Candace had relished this war, delighting as opponents were vanquished and humiliated. "I wanted to be ready to leap into the fray myself and do battle with the boys," she writes, ". . . so caught up was I in the drama of the competition, the lust to win."

Candace was Snyder's perfect lieutenant—"my little girl," he called her—until the day she refused to do his bidding, when she chose herself over him. "Candace was brilliant, passionate, fearless, and bold. Sol said she was one of the smartest people he'd ever met," reflects Edythe London, who began studying under Snyder the year Candace left for the NIMH. "I would imagine that she fueled him." Yet the relationship between a mentor and mentee is like a complex love affair that often ends poorly, with a protégé demanding credit while a mentor resents his pupil's lack of gratitude. "Sol and Candace had the classic mentor-mentee relationship. She worshipped him and he probably loved her too, until she was fighting him."

Candace and Snyder's 1973 paper on the opiate receptor would become one of the most cited in history, with more than four thousand citations, where an average paper might receive fifty. Regardless, the scientific community was aghast that Candace would confront her mentor in public. In doing so, she wasn't just airing dirty laundry; she was exposing the petty rivalries and messy inner workings of a field ostensibly governed by reason. It was nothing short of disgraceful.

So in 1979, when the scandal-averse Nobel committee chose to venerate a separate set of male scientists, Candace was blamed for spurring a public fracas that mortified Snyder and effectively disqualified him and the Aberdeen team from receiving the Nobel Prize. The backlash she received was swift and lethal. Candace was blackballed by her scientific family and branded a self-serving troublemaker, the "scarlet woman of neuroscience"—a reputation that would plague her for years to come.

CHAPTER FOUR

POISON PILL

ANDACE'S TRAILBLAZING PATH WAS FRAUGHT WITH BARRIERS NO MAN OF HER generation would encounter. In the 1980s, female scientists at the NIH were objects of scorn, particularly if they had children. To be admitted into the vaunted intramural program was particularly rare for women, and it meant that Candace was fighting for the same titles and resources as male peers.

"If you're a woman working in my lab or a lab assistant, that's fine. But when you got tenure and were competing against men, you're a crazy bitch," says Betsy Parker, a fellow PhD in the NIH intramural program who was awarded tenure shortly after Candace. "If you had kids, then they thought you were a real witch: 'You should be home!'" Most coworkers were men with stay-at-home wives or wives who worked in distinctly subordinate roles.

Parker, like Candace, had been the senior scientist recruited to the NIH who greased the wheels for her husband's appointment, yet colleagues assumed she was a charity hire. Male associates were horrified when she attended an important meeting at a superior's office three days after giving birth to her second son, and when Parker applied to lead a neuropsychology section, her lab chief rejected her petition on the grounds that it would "give the guys castration anxiety."

"I said, 'I'm the only one who's published in this area. I'm the only one who's known nationally and internationally!'" she recounts. "He said the guys didn't like me." Finally, when Parker was awarded tenure, jealous male peers spread rumors that she'd slept her way to the top. It simply wasn't possible for a woman to have made it on her own; if she'd succeeded, it was only after spreading her legs for an influential boss. "It wasn't true," Parker says, "but it was perception."

When asked about the Lasker scandal, Parker insists that it wasn't a scandal at all, but rather a gross injustice. The true scandal, she says, was the well-known pattern of behavior that enabled male colleagues to steal credit for women's work. Whenever a female scientist generated a brilliant idea, her male counterparts assumed it was the brainchild of whatever man she was working with, and he would inevitably receive recognition. "We used to call it the 'Old Fart Effect,'" she says, "and Candace addressed it, so good for her."

When considering bias in science and healthcare, it is telling that the NIH required research studies to include women and minorities in their study populations only in 1986, and it wasn't until the early 1990s that policy revisions ensured their inclusion. Only white men's needs were considered worthy of study and treatment, and this prejudice was reflected in the hierarchy at the National Institutes of Health.

According to a 2022 study published in *Nature*, this inequity persists even forty years later. After reviewing some 9,700 research teams—including information on payments and job titles for all researchers working on a given grant, as well as the credit each scientist was awarded on related papers and patents—researchers found that women are 13 percent less likely to be listed on articles and 58 percent less likely to be included on patents than their male collaborators, controlling for factors such as seniority. The more cited or influential a paper, the less likely women scientists are to be named; on papers with twenty-five or more citations, women are 20 percent more likely to be excluded from authorship, as rules for credit allocation remain vague. Therefore, recognition is determined by senior investigators, who are, for the most part, male. As in Candace's day, female scientists tend to receive attribution only when it's conferred by their male superiors, and women continue to be shamed and vilified for highlighting discrimination.

Candace paid a hefty price, as her rabble-rousing reputation dominated her time at the NIH. Senior administrators who controlled funding and conferred prizes weren't apt to acknowledge women in the first place, much less a female firebrand. Plus, Sol Snyder retained close ties with top brass and had pulled strings to get Candace and Agu hired, so his protégé was viewed as churlish. "The perception was: *How dare she?* How dare she rock the establishment this way?" Parker continues, stressing that infighting for the Lasker Award, Candace had put her career on the line. "The way people talked about her after that was very dismissive—like 'Candace, she's a problem.' Never that she's a great scientist."

Despite the blowback she received, Candace continued to use her platform to advocate for women's health. She loved the limelight and was, in fact, a reporter's dream, firing off provocative quotes, such as: "Don't get me wrong, I like men—but in their place, which is the bedroom. Let them out, and they start wars." Much to the consternation of male superiors, she also breastfed her babies in the front row of scientific conferences and, because she'd hated being sedated for Evan's birth, became a vocal proponent of natural childbirth.

A 1979 *Washington Post Magazine* profile describes a scene in which Candace and NIH colleagues discuss a journal article that suggests that natural childbirth may be better for an infant than accepted obstetric practices of the time, which included the liberal use of drugs. When a peer notes that the paper's female author appeared "abrasive" before a Food and Drug Administration (FDA) panel, Candace counters, "There is another side to this. Many of us think she is some kind of saint for what she has been willing to go through to bring this information to light." While Candace's perspective on healthcare undoubtedly helped women overall, and while the publicity she garnered shed light on the field's inequities for women, such public declarations rankled her male bosses.

Calling herself a "New Wave" scientist, Candace rejected Snyder's dog-eat-dog management style in favor of openness and intellectual autonomy. Instead of competition, she preached collaboration, promising her top-notch underlings that wonders, as well as credit and prizes, awaited if they stuck together and played as a team. Hers was a decidedly feminine, and feminist, mode of leadership. Having faced bigotry herself, Candace also fostered diversity and a sense of democracy in her lab. She made it a point to hire women and people of color, knowing all too well that she'd recruit better talent, as marginalized groups must work twice as hard and be twice as good to be recognized. Candace intuited long before studies proved it that varying perspectives produce more creative outcomes.

As a manager, Candace emoted in zealous rants rather than threatening fury, and she made no attempts at manly gravitas. Somehow, there was an innocence to her transgressions. Her tantrums were like the flailing of a capricious child and were matched by an endearing wonder about the world, a pure passion for discovery, and a total lack of pretension or self-consciousness. Even at work, Candace ate with her hands, licked chocolate off her fingers, and painted rainbows on her nails and office walls.

"She was into 'joy of life' kind of things," reflects Miles Herkenham, her frequent collaborator who went on to become senior investigator in

the Section on Functional Neuroanatomy of the Laboratory of Cellular and Molecular Regulation at the NIH. "I gravitate toward people
who are positive because it counters my dour mood. I need people to
boost me, and she did that in a big way. She even came to my softball
games. She was a cheerleader for everyone." While others held grudges,
Candace overflowed with maternal warmth and forgiveness; although
she'd been burned by Snyder, she tried on multiple occasions to make
amends with him and was quick to apologize when she offended others. "That universal benevolence was always there."

Far from being a "science nun," Candace had chosen a complex
existence with many moving parts, especially having had children well
ahead of her peers. Presaging current debate, she was adamant that to
succeed professionally, women needed help at home. Thus, she surrounded herself with people who would scaffold her mission, including Agu, whom the Beebes credit with buoying Candace, tempering
her extremes, and paving her way to greatness. "Candy wouldn't be
who she was if not for Agu Pert. He's a remarkable man, and everyone
should have a husband like him," says her cousin Nancy Morris. "Agu
became the love of our family. We're all still close."

When Candace enrolled as a twenty-four-year-old doctoral candidate at Hopkins, Mildred and Bob became frequent visitors at
Edgewood Arsenal and Agu stepped in as Evan's primary caregiver,
shouldering responsibilities so that Candace could focus on her studies. "It would be unreasonable for me to expect her to cook a meal when
she came back from graduate school at 7 p.m.," he says matter-of-factly.
"I wasn't a great cook, but I picked up those skills." Asked whether he
ever grew aggrieved by his wife's external commitments, Agu under-
scores that his own formidable, resilient mother had raised him to
believe marriage should be egalitarian, and that she and his stepfather
were true partners. As evidence, Agu notes that the Estonian language

lacks distinct words for "husband" and "wife," eschewing gender roles by referring to both as "helpmate." "That's the way I was brought up," he says. "I think Candace and I worked well as a team."

While Candace was a stereotypical adoring Jewish mother, to say she needed a helpmate was an understatement. Mildred's doting had a downside, and by the time Candace had a family of her own, she'd never learned how to keep a home or perform the basic functions of adulthood. She would leave a trail of clothes or food exploded on the counter, as though Mildred were following behind to tidy up. And after the opiate receptor discovery, Mildred began accompanying Candace to conferences and speaking engagements to dress her lest, as one cousin puts it, "she'd have a boob hanging out and not think anything of it." Even Grandma Rose would regularly clean Candace's home and care for Evan.

Candace also engaged her sisters to assist, and during the summer of 1971, when Deane was in high school, she and her friend moved into Candace and Agu's apartment at Edgewood Arsenal to perform domestic duties. "I was also Candace's personal slave," Deane says. "Candy was off in Baltimore and Agu was at the base, so we were like the mothers." Deane and her friend cared for Evan and prepared meals, and at night they'd socialize with locals, smoking pot and attending concerts with hippies. Mildred and Bob never would have allowed such behavior at their home on Long Island, so Deane saw it as a win.

One night, Deane and her friend were invited inside a laundromat by Deborah Stokes, a recent high school graduate who worked there and feared the young women would be assaulted outside in this rough part of town. Before long, Deane learned that Stokes was living in a one-bedroom apartment in the projects with her alcoholic, mentally ill mother and four sisters, three of whom she was raising. Her father had left them two years before, so Stokes was supporting her family with meager wages. Knowing that Candace would need a nanny for Evan come fall, Deane brought Stokes to interview for the job.

Stokes remembers being struck by Candace and Agu's apartment, which was bright and overstuffed with art, including a large canvas on which Candace had pressed her naked body after rolling in a can of paint. Prior to meeting the Beebes, Agu's command of aesthetics had been confined to the mass-produced Italian oil paintings of pastoral scenes that lined the walls of his parents' home, as well as every other home in their neighborhood. But Bob had shepherded Candace and Agu to gallery openings and to the Museum of Modern Art to view the work of modern masters such as Dalí and Calder, which informed the couple's taste in décor. Their home was a bohemian oasis amid the "army slum," as Candace called it, and Stokes was keen to stay.

Typical of the Rosenberg clan, Candace adopted people and took them under her wing, and Stokes credits her with shaping the trajectory of her life. She'd never met a progressive freethinker like Candace, a woman who took up space and seemed entirely indifferent to fitting in. While other army wives sprayed their hair into beehive helmets, Candace embraced her wild, natural curls and didn't shave her legs. She was mouthy, opinionated, warm, and wild. "She really let her freak flag fly," Stokes says. "I swear, they broke the mold with her." Candace saw Stokes's potential, mentored her, and introduced her to *Ms.* magazine, guiding Stokes toward feminism.

Stokes, whom Candace later appointed Evan's godmother, had never imagined a healthy, equal partnership, much less seen one up close, and she marveled at Candace and Agu's marriage. Candace was a playful, loving mother whom Evan adored. Each morning, she scrambled brown eggs for him and then left her son's care to Agu and Stokes. During the five years Stokes watched Evan, becoming part of the family, Candace helped her get scholarships, first to community college and then to a four-year university, where Stokes followed her mentor into biology. "Candace was like a big sister," Stokes says. "With her, friends became family and family was everything."

While Candace prioritized relationships, as with Deborah Stokes, her connections often had a transactional quality, cultivated to serve her purpose. She was a master at bending others to her will and cagey about favors, casting her requests as beneficial for the counterparty. For instance, once Deane had graduated from college, Candace tried to convince her sister to spend a summer working as a nanny for an important Italian colleague with whom she wanted to cement a relationship. "I was like, 'I don't want to sleep in some kid's room as a babysitter. I have my own life,'" Deane scoffs. "It wasn't for me. It was to help *her*. With Candace, it was always about *her* life."

Having seen women sidelined, Candace advocated for her own needs and counseled other working mothers to prioritize themselves. When her Hopkins colleague Anne Young learned that she was pregnant during her residency in neurology, Candace called and said, "Anne, let me tell you how to deal with this," Young recalls. "Hire someone to live in your house and be there whenever you want and pay them. Even if it's one whole person's salary, it's worth it. Someone's got to take care of the kids, and that's the only way you'll get through working when your husband is too."

Following her own guidance, when Candace and Agu moved to Bethesda to work at the NIH, they hired an older nanny/housekeeper from El Salvador to care for Evan and their daughter, Vanessa, who had been born in April 1975, just after Candace earned her PhD. Though the family ate dinner together, Candace and Agu routinely brought work home, and evenings were dominated by scientific debate. "Both of us should have been more involved with the children," Agu reflects. "Our lives revolved pretty much around our work, and that's the regret I have."

Yet Candace never separated work from her personal life; each aspect of existence bled into the next, as evidenced when her beloved father got sick. In 1980, Bob was diagnosed with small-cell lung cancer, a deadly carcinoma Candace understood all too well, as its rapidly dividing cells were full of the peptides, or types of proteins that bind selectively to specific receptors, that she'd been studying. Immediately, Candace leveraged her expertise in peptide chemistry and called the top small-cell clinician at the NIH's National Cancer Institute (NCI) to strike a deal. In exchange for allowing her father entry into current trials, though his age exceeded the protocols' limit, the doctor secured Candace's help identifying exactly which neuropeptides were being secreted by small-cell cancer cells. This would lend insight into how and why these cells multiply, which could lead to better treatments, if not a cure.

Candace quickly discovered that each cancer cell line she'd received from the NCI's lab was marked by a high level of the peptide bombesin, which meant that bombesin was driving small cells' persistent growth. If she could determine how bombesin worked, then perhaps she could locate an antagonist to block the cells' proliferation in time to save her father. Science was urgent and personal then, and Candace provided a glimmer of hope during a devastating time for her family. "My mother told me stories about their love, how when my uncle was sick Candy got in bed with him in the hospital and held him all night," says Nancy Morris. "He was so proud of her."

When Bob died within a year, Candace cajoled her mother to move from Long Island to Maryland to help raise her grandchildren. Mildred insisted on renting her own apartment, however, and ventured to establish an independent life as a young widow of sixty, making new friends and securing a part-time job at a children's clothing store. Still, much of her time and energy was spent as Candace's unpaid nanny and personal assistant, running household errands and shuttling children to school, sports, activities, and appointments. This meant that Candace's brood received the same favored status she'd been granted as a child, as Mildred saw her other grandchildren far less often. "Candy was kind and generous, but also very persuasive," Deane says. "Whatever was right for Candy, she wanted everyone to do. You name it, she wanted it to be her way."

While Candace cast herself as a champion of women, she tended to put her personal interests above all. At both home and work, she claimed the center of attention and, try as she might to curb her competitive instincts, her ambition remained a driving force. Candace was known to engineer situations to her advantage, and sometimes she didn't play fair. She would initiate races in a swimming pool, saying, "Ready, set . . . ," and then suddenly she'd be two strokes ahead on "Go!" She even schooled her children in this survival-of-the-fittest mindset, beating them at checkers and Scrabble and howling, "No mercy! Do better next time!"

Candace also locked horns with Agu, who, notwithstanding his unwavering support during the Lasker controversy, felt eclipsed by her time in the limelight after discovering the opiate receptor. "I was quite proud of Candace, but as always there's a little competition and jealousy," he explains. "There was some resentment maybe on my part, which increased in subsequent years. That was my fault, anyway; I wasn't as aggressive in promoting myself." Still, the press Candace received—touting her first as a prodigy and then as a feminist heroine—seemed to go to her head, swelling an already robust ego. Many observed that she also treated Agu like hired help.

Some question Candace's commitment to feminism and believe that she cultivated female journalists in the wake of the Lasker flap and founded Women in Neuroscience, a network of female support, simply to aid her agenda. "Candace didn't take up the fight for women. She took up the fight for herself," says her Hopkins colleague Edythe London. "Sol was a major careerist, but she'd also bought into it, especially if she didn't mention Avram Goldstein's work [in her paper]. She just didn't like the corruption when it affected her."

Moreover, according to her Hopkins lab mate Anne Young, Candace could be ruthless in asserting her advantage, even over other women. Young recalls that shortly after graduate school, she and Candace reunited at a conference and began discussing the autoradiography method Candace had learned from Mike Kuhar and was employing at the NIH with Miles Herkenham to map receptors with neural pathways. Young says that the process Candace had used at the NIH was cumbersome and inexact, while the technique Young had refined in her lab at the University of Michigan was swift and precise, yielding loads of quantitative detail. Since Young had just submitted a paper on the topic to *Science*, she was happy to share her approach with Candace.

Soon after, however, Young was stunned to receive two divergent reviews on her *Science* paper; one was glowing, while the other was indifferent enough that the paper was declined. Young instantly deduced that Candace had written the lukewarm review to sabotage her and "skim the cream"—a suspicion confirmed when Young received the latest issue of *Nature*, whose cover advertised an article by Candace featuring a radiant, rainbow-colored slice of brain analyzed using Young's methodology. Incensed, Young called the *Science* editor to see if she'd been snookered. "The editor takes a look and says, 'Your paper will be in next week,'" she says. "She got my paper rejected, then took our method! We were friends. Why would she do that to me?"

To answer Young's question, one must consider the backbiting cultures of both Johns Hopkins and the National Institutes of Health, as well as the importance of intrinsic morality in matters of service and healing. We, as a society, want to believe that those bound by the Hippocratic oath ("first, do no harm") are altruistic and driven by pure intentions. But how many doctors feel a desire to heal that overshadows their urge to control or exert a godlike power to save lives? How many bureaucrats value assisting others over their capacity to influence or rule? How much do motives matter if one's deeds aid humanity regardless?

The NIH was fashioned on the lofty premise that clinical advances are fast-tracked when superb scientists are given free rein to explore. Highlighting its academic nature, the NIH's sprawling headquarters is called a "campus" where, in return for capped pay, intramural researchers pursue their interests unhindered by commercial constraints. Yet despite the security this federally funded intellectual playground provides, doctors and scientists remain subject to the same enmity and greed that blight other industries. They are not a league of saints.

It is said that in academia "the knives are so sharp because the stakes are so low." In an environment of scarcity where researchers earn modest wages and vie for meager grants, one's status depends almost entirely on acknowledgment by one's peers. Scientific papers—which were never meant to be used as currency, but rather to convey discoveries, replications, and validations—have become the sole mark of distinction for which researchers are rewarded for being first and right. Frenzied disputes over credit are common, as defective incentive structures perpetuate dysfunctional behavior. Researchers eviscerate each other's studies and grant applications rather than helping refine ideas, and infighting lends a sense of superiority, as scientists cast themselves as gatekeepers of truth.

Candace subscribed to this construct. She had shown herself to be an opportunist as avid as Sol Snyder, but her steamrolling lacked finesse, as she brazenly took down anyone, male or female, who stood between her and her goal. By her own admission, she had "gotten good at swimming with sharks," relishing the cutthroat cultures of Hopkins and the NIH so long as they propelled her success. If this was how men "played the game," she reasoned, then why should she be different?

Yet Candace was held to different standards because of her gender. Historically, with men it is results that are prioritized, while women are scrutinized for their motivations. Powerful men like Snyder are revered even when driven by ego, particularly if the outcome of their actions is positive for society. However, when women attain power, they must evince virtue or risk being shunned.

As a result, Candace and women of her generation faced a double bind. When presented with generations of a dominant white, patriarchal hegemony in which brute displays of force were synonymous with strong leadership, they replicated this behavior to compete. But while cruelty or subversion in white men is understood and excused as linked to their talents—after all, they *have to* be tough to succeed—society somehow condemns such conduct in others. When women and people of color adopt identical tactics, they are seldom given the benefit of the doubt, and their brilliance is overshadowed by their perceived malevolence. Displays of power inevitably prove a poison pill.

What, then, are the consequences of an irreverent, morally ambiguous woman fearlessly trying to change the world? A feminist lens suggests that the quality of Candace's work was largely irrelevant to the way she was received. It didn't matter if Candace was a genius or if her work surpassed that of male peers. By jockeying and vying for power with men, she was seen as unnatural, and so was spurned.

CHAPTER FIVE

"THE CRAZIES"

ESPITE THE DISCRIMINATION CANDACE FACED, SHE ALSO UNDERMINED HERself, as she seemed simultaneously aware of her impetuous conduct yet incapable of modulating it.

Like her free-spirit parents, Candace drew people in and pissed people off with her lack of boundaries. While she was staying with her cousins, her behavior included meditating and doing yoga nude before the living room window. Sometimes, without permission, she'd try to nurse her cousins' babies, intending it as an act of love to cement the family bond.

Candace also took liberties with strangers, channeling her emotions freely as they arose. Once, while standing in line at a pharmacy, she turned to a sullen couple behind her and scolded the husband, "Don't frown! You have a great wife standing there. Kiss her right now!" While visiting Disneyland for a conference, she grabbed a grumpy guest at the bar, pulled him onto the dance floor, spun him around, and then made him dance with his wife. Believing she could help people surmount self-imposed limitations, Candace perpetually meddled in others' business and propounded her often unwanted views. She was a disruptor in every area of life.

"When a person is like that, you're always on guard wondering what they're going to throw out and what you'll have to deal with," says her childhood friend Nancy Marriott. "In some ways, she reminded me of Lucille Ball in the way she was daffy. She was a woman unwilling to be put down, suppressed, shackled, or gagged."

Friends and colleagues note with alternating affection and derision that Candace was unabashedly unique, a larger-than-life magnet for drama, someone who loved to shock others and to flaunt her body. She reveled in being the "sexy scientist," overturning stereotypes of female researchers as prudes in Coke-bottle glasses. Even in graduate school, while most women wore conservative suits or jeans with work shirts, Candace sported flimsy, revealing dresses, sometimes without underwear, and was known to swan around, teasing men. "A lot of guys would see this behavior and say, 'Better for me not to be here,'" says Anne Young. Like her parents, Candace also vamped for Halloween, but her costumes boasted a sexual flair. Generally, she favored "slutty witch" and "slutty nurse" outfits, yet at the height of the toxic shock syndrome epidemic associated with some types of tampons, she arrived at a party for NIH employees dressed as a bloody Tampax.

Needless to say, this approach didn't fly in the workplace, and coworkers were appalled when Candace sunbathed nude in public or exposed her body on a whim. Her colleague Edythe London recalls that after a conference in Puerto Rico sponsored by the American College of Neuropsychopharmacology, Candace wanted to go swimming one last time before departing for the airport. Instead of allotting time to change, however, she chose to strip in a cab in traffic, mooning coworkers and people in surrounding vehicles. "Candace was a force," London says. "Always thinking, always with a spark, and very outrageous."

Not all of Candace's female peers were as generous, as many women who worked overtime to earn respect and break glass ceilings found her exhibitionism unsettling. Lydia Temoshok, a clinical psychologist who was then a professor of medicine at the Institute of Human Virology at the University of Maryland, Baltimore School of Medicine, recalls that when she first met Candace at a conference, Candace was wearing fishnet stockings, a short, tight skirt, and a low-cut shirt that left little to the imagination. "She was so confident going up to the podium, but I thought, 'Why would you do that, even if you had the best body in the world?'" Temoshok says. "She set herself up not to be accepted professionally." However, when the two women began talking, Candace understood concepts that others failed to grasp and was complimentary about her paper, so Temoshok accepted her as a professional.

While colleagues delighted in Candace's spontaneity, they also say that her "loose cannon" stunts could be alarming. Along with her body, she made no attempt to hide her penchant for illegal substances, regularly smoking weed on the steps of the NIH. At a winter conference on brain research in Colorado, she baked hash brownies at one of her infamous parties and when they caught fire, filling her condo with smoke, she handed the tray to firefighters at the scene: "Here, have some!"

And once, while working with Miles Herkenham, whom Candace unabashedly called a "hunk," she spilled a dish of tritium, a radioactive isotope of hydrogen, on the laboratory floor. "It's a big deal," he says, "and she was always in a hurry." Herkenham had been trained and licensed to work with radioactive substances, but Candace had not. Yet instead of abiding by protocol, she let out a bloodcurdling scream and ran into the hallway to find a janitor. "I just saw a cockroach!" she cried. "I spilled and need you to clean it up!" Compared with other types of radioactive materials, tritium is largely harmless, but Candace always considered herself above the rules.

Herkenham, who went on to discover the cannabinoid receptor, insists that Candace wasn't a crusader for women and was thwarted not because of her gender but because she was outlandish, unseemly, and unable to foresee the consequences of her actions. Though Herkenham's boss—"a straitlaced white guy neurophysiologist, but they were all white guys back then"—originally encouraged him to work with Candace and was enamored of their progress, he came to find her escapades distasteful. "She was so flamboyant that she put people off. She caused schisms. People would say, 'I don't want to deal with this' and turn her off," he says. "It's hard to distinguish that from sexism. It was her as an individual, not her as a woman."

Many colleagues bristled at Candace's brash, mercurial style, and her collaborations at the NIH were as fraught as they were frequent. She'd even made a foe of the lab director with whom she'd worked on small-cell carcinoma when her father was ill. She knew that the scrappy "game" of science required researchers to claim credit by dribbling data into as many papers as possible, thus increasing their chances for citations and awards. However, without buy-in from her partner on the project, Candace had front-loaded all their data into a single paper in *Science*, squandering additional opportunities for recognition. Her peer was further incensed when her lab extended their joint research and published a separate paper in *The Lancet* without him.

Candace insists that her intentions were good. With her father dying during the final months of her third pregnancy, she'd lost her taste for blood. Instead of wanting to best her peers, she'd begun to see the human side of research and the people she could help. She hadn't managed to save Bob, but she thought that by cramming one paper full of data she could move the field closer to a cure. Even so, the cancer lab director felt undermined, and after that he wanted nothing to do with her.

What's worse, colleagues say that Candace flouted the scientific method, which requires a researcher to make every effort to disprove hypotheses. Instead, she performed only experiments to buttress her ideas and prove her hypotheses, prompting Herkenham to joke that Candace never let data get between her and a good story. She didn't falsify or manipulate data, he says, but rather saw what she wanted to see and cherry-picked to make her point.

Herkenham hit a proverbial wall when he and Candace were collaborating on a draft of a paper and she wrote something "absolutely crazy" in the discussion section, causing him to insist that, as phrased, her hypothesis could not be tested. "The poor woman who was our first author was ready to shoot herself," he remembers. "At some point, I had to pull away. That was one of the last papers I did with her because we didn't have the same language." Though they remained lifelong friends, and Herkenham even married his second wife in 1997 in Candace's backyard, he avoided broaching science with her thereafter.

Like Herkenham, Agu grew frustrated by the very traits that drew him to Candace. He found it exhausting to live in the state of mayhem she courted, but when Agu failed to match Candace's ferment or fury, she called him conservative and pessimistic; even small things like his mustache, which he'd had since age twenty, were the source of endless debate. "Candace was an amazing person, but not easy to live with," Agu says. "Maybe I was too boring for her."

At Fort Sam and Edgewood Arsenal, Agu had enjoyed Candace's irreverence and never minded that she didn't mix with other military wives, as he too found their white-glove traditions archaic and affected. He'd never been attracted to uptight, subservient women who adhered to gender norms, and he hadn't even blinked when Candace baked anatomically correct gingerbread cookies for a Christmas party hosted by his boss, a Southern Baptist colonel. Agu had already become branch chief of his unit and was planning to leave the military to work at the NIMH, but he recalls a long silence after the treats were unwrapped and "these Southern Baptists fell off their chairs."

Though Agu wasn't directly penalized for the scandals caused by his wife, her professional battles proved grueling for their family. As the stress of Candace's workplace and Bob's death took its toll, she became increasingly volatile, and soon it was clear that her emotional swings veered well outside the norm. Aside from her college hospitalization, Candace had never shown signs of depression or psychosis. Primarily, she was hypomanic, a state characterized by supercharged energy during which the "afflicted" can be remarkably fruitful. Indeed, she went undiagnosed by both her NIMH boss, Fred Goodwin, and her lab chief and administrator, Steve Paul, who were both psychiatrists with expertise in bipolar disorder.

"I never saw her floridly manic. She had bouts of hypomania, as do some of the more creative people in the world," says Paul, who spent eighteen years at the NIH as a laboratory/branch chief and as scientific director of the NIMH. "Occasionally, there was a pretty intense element to her passion, but I can't say yea or nay. As a shrink, I'm not sure it would be appropriate."

Here, Paul references the work of Kay Redfield Jamison, a professor of psychiatry at the Johns Hopkins University School of Medicine who coauthored with Fred Goodwin the medical text *Manic-Depressive Illness* and has written extensively about her own experience being bipolar. In her 1993 book *Touched with Fire: Manic-Depressive Illness and the Artistic Temperament*, Jamison explores the link between hypomania and intellectual or artistic achievement, arguing that hypomania increases the "fluency, rapidity, and flexibility of thought on the one hand, and the ability to combine ideas or categories of thought in order to form new and original connections on the other." After conceding bipolar disorder's obvious downsides, including suicidal tendencies, Jamison asks, "Who would *not* want an illness that has among its symptoms elevated and expansive mood, inflated self-esteem, abundance of energy, less need for sleep, intensified sexuality and—most germane to our argument here—'sharpened and unusually creative thinking' and 'increased productivity'?"

Agu concurs, acknowledging that Candace did some of her most inspired, original thinking while hypomanic. He notes that Sir Isaac Newton likely suffered from bipolar disorder and psychosis, penning delusional letters to family and friends while inventing calculus and deciphering the force of universal gravity. And Beethoven and Winston Churchill used their manic stretches to compose back-to-back verses and books, respectively, before falling into dark depressions. Similarly, for a period of seven or eight years, Candace flourished in this state.

Until the Lasker Award, that is. To cope with her distress over Snyder's betrayal, Candace attended Erhard Seminars Training (EST), a two-weekend, sixty-hour course of guided personal transformation meant to free participants from negative behaviors and encourage accountability for one's life. There, she felt a deep awareness of raw emotions and a moment of transcendent consciousness. "God is in the frontal cortex," she later concluded. "As the part of the brain that gives us the ability to decide and plan for the future, to make changes, to exert control over our lives, the frontal cortex seemed to me to be the only way I could explain what I had seen and experienced. It seemed to me to be the God within each of us."

While Candace acknowledged the food and sleep deprivation she endured and that she'd struggled to integrate the experience, Agu says it precipitated her next psychotic break. "EST is very destructive to a person who's fragile. It's very harsh and tears a person down completely with sleep deprivation," he asserts. "They berate you. A person who is fragile can be damaged." When Candace returned home, she began crawling on the floor and clawing at her husband's face, claiming he was the devil. "Her brain was fried. She was delusional."

At a loss, Agu called Sol Snyder for help. Candace's mentor had instigated her trauma, but he was also a psychiatrist operating at the forefront of his field and could recommend a course of treatment. On Snyder's advice, Agu drove Candace in the middle of the night to Adventist Hospital in Langley Park, where she remained sedated and dosed with antipsychotics for three weeks. She was clinically depressed for several months afterward and prescribed the heavy antidepressants she'd been investigating in her lab. In a painful twist on the catch-phrase "research is *me*-search," just as Candace was working at the National Institute of Mental Health to understand and treat mental illness, she was suffering a cycle of bipolar disorder.

Though Agu confided in the couple's branch chief, at the time the stigma around mental illness was so severe that even doctors on the cutting edge of psychiatry and psychopharmacology were loath to discuss it. "Candace couldn't afford to get treatment with bipolar. They'd kick her out!" says Betsy Parker, her NIH peer. "She probably didn't want to accept it herself, but professionally she could never have admitted to mental illness. Of all the fields you would think there would be acceptance, the people studying mental health were terrible about it, the most judgmental."

Anne Young agrees that any hint of emotional instability was, and arguably still is, the kiss of death for women. In the 1970s and '80s, even doctors went to great lengths to hide chinks in their mental and emotional armor. "No one saw a psychiatrist," she says. "It meant you were crazy." So, upon returning to work, Candace labored to conceal her debility. In a 1979 *Washington Post* magazine profile that chronicles Candace and Agu's search for therapies for schizophrenia and depression, she depicts their mission flippantly as "trying to cure the crazies." A year prior, she was quoted in a separate article as saying, "People will tell you the most intimate details of their sex lives—I mean strangers on a plane. But if someone has a brother or a sister or a husband who has cracked up, that's a deep dark secret."

All the while, Candace was keeping a secret of her own: that mental illness ran in her family. According to Beebe lore, Bob's mother "took to her room" to escape a loveless marriage, and while Bob had been hospitalized for PTSD after World War II, he also suffered from bipolar disorder. He was known to stay up all night cooking or wander into the backyard, place his false teeth in his bathrobe pocket, and smoke Camel cigarettes down to nubs. Mildred would call, "Bob, what are you doing?" and he'd respond, "I'm thinking!"

Candace's middle sister, Wynne, had been diagnosed with bipolar disorder as well. After studying fine arts at Indiana University, she'd earned a master's degree at Oberlin University and become an art restorer at the Metropolitan Museum of Art in Manhattan. After her first breakdown in 1972, she'd retreated to Bob and Mildred's home on Long Island and then, without warning, made her way to Edgewood Arsenal, where Candace and Agu spent days nursing her back to relative health. Once Wynne returned to her parents' house, however, she became paranoid and dissociated and was hospitalized again.

Now, Candace and Agu's relationship was deteriorating, in part because of her condition. Though Agu raised eyebrows by embarking on a relationship with an NIH postdoc fifteen years his junior, Candace had been courting extramarital affairs for years. Of course, Agu knew that his wife was cheeky and beguiling, but he'd dismissed her coquetry as playful. At the NIH, the couple worked together closely in offices separated only by a thin wall, so he isn't sure exactly when her cheating started. Yet he suspects that while he was in denial, their friends and coworkers knew Candace was "promiscuous."

Even before Candace had discovered the opiate receptor, Snyder had sent her and Anne Young to Nashville for two months to a prestigious neuropharmacology seminar taught by leaders in the field. Students— about seventy in total, fewer than ten of whom were women—were all rising stars, and they often networked after hours in bars and bluegrass clubs. There, Candace began sidling up to men, though she knew Agu was coming to visit. He and Young's husband had planned to join their wives for a quick road trip to the Great Smoky Mountains, but when Agu arrived, he found Candace in another man's room. "Maybe she was trying to make him mad," says Young, who overheard the fiery battle that ensued. "What was she doing in some guy's room? Her life was complicated. It was very hard."

After years of training as a neurologist, Young, who went on to become chief of the neurology service at Massachusetts General Hospital and a professor at Harvard Medical School, recognized in retrospect that Candace was likely bipolar, so she made a conscious effort to forgive her for stealing her autoradiography technique. "I really thought she was sick, so why should I get all worked up?" Young continues. "It was so interesting to see her in action. Her mind, her creative mind, was incredibly rich. She was always coming up with new things, but when it came to evaluating certain parts of her life, she really had trouble."

By 1982, Candace and Agu had formally separated in a split everyone agrees was ugly. The couple's third pregnancy hadn't helped to solidify their bond, as they'd hoped, and Candace's most recent relationship with an NIH colleague had sparked a bitter, public clash. Eventually, Agu came to view his wife's heightened sexuality as a symptom of her illness, but still he was crushed, especially because their own connection was so passionate. "Candace and I had a very good sexual relationship, but it was never enough for her," he says. "I didn't have an affair. Candace had affairs. It wasn't an easy thing for me to process and I'm still trying to come to grips with it, why I put up with it."

The couple found a mediator in Alexandria, Virginia, and paid $300 each for a divorce that was, in the end, remarkably amicable considering the bluster of their initial breakup. Candace and Agu still had deep feelings for each other, and they left the courthouse grief-stricken about their inability to sustain a union. Though they had agreed to an equal division of assets and joint custody of their children, the latter proved impractical when Agu moved to a townhouse thirty minutes away. While Evan was a teenager, Vanessa was only seven years old and Brandon was an infant; the children needed stability and routine, so they came to live primarily in Bethesda with Candace and spent alternating weekends, as well as one full month each summer, with Agu.

Unlike her Hopkins counterpart Kay Redfield Jamison, Candace continued to deny her illness and came to hate the very drugs she was researching, as she felt they dulled her edge. "She never admitted she was ill, which is a characteristic of the disorder, saying, 'It's not me, it's you. You're the one who has the problem,'" Agu says. Though Candace had psychotic episodes every seven to eight years, in between them she was undeniably prolific. Much of her life was spent in the hypomanic state that allowed her to prosper, and one is left to wonder, as she did, whether medication would have blunted her genius. Was madness the price of carrying a torch to illuminate humankind?

CHAPTER SIX

BODYMIND

For the first time in her life, Candace found herself the primary caretaking parent without a daily helpmate. Though she mourned her marriage, she wasn't prone to let grass grow under her feet.

Shortly after her separation from Agu, when she wandered into a bar just off the NIH campus with baby Brandon strapped to her chest, Candace wasn't looking for new love. But as she took a seat beside a handsome young postdoc, she felt flattered that he recognized her. Michael Ruff had seen her in a science documentary, discussing how endorphins from the testes cause orgasmic spasms in the vas deferens, the duct that transports sperm from the testicles to the urethra for ejaculation, and he seemed eager to unpack her findings. This was geeky flirting at its best.

However, the instant Candace learned that Michael and his friend Rick Weber were immunologists, "she sucked us dry," he says, interrogating them about their chosen field of study. Candace's interest in immunology had begun more than a year before, when her father was diagnosed with small-cell lung cancer and she'd collaborated with a researcher from the National Cancer Institute. Though Bob had relapsed and died, she saw through her grief a silver lining in this interdisciplinary approach to research, as a cross-sector methodology yielded better results.

In the tradition of her scientific bloodline, Candace had already benefitted from a curiosity that extended well beyond the confines of her specialty, and her ability to bridge divides and make connections had sparked her grand innovation. So, similar to the handshake agreement she'd made with the cancer lab director, she arranged to teach Michael and Rick Weber brain receptor science if they'd teach her immunology. There, in the bar, Candace and Michael launched a personal and professional partnership that would last the rest of her lifetime.

Shortly after their barroom powwow, Weber discovered a shocking article by Ed Blalock, a graduate school classmate who claimed to have found a type of white blood cells called lymphocytes that secreted endorphins. Of course, they knew that endorphins were the peptides that bind to the opiate receptor in the brain, but if Blalock was correct, did this mean that there were opiate receptors on immune cell surfaces too? With her underlings' assistance, Candace designed assays to test this hypothesis, and once again her findings exceeded expectations, demonstrating receptors on immune cells for nearly every peptide or drug identified in the brain.

This meant that the brain was communicating with the immune system, but Candace wanted to know if the conversation was reciprocal. Could the immune system also "speak" to the brain? The next logical step was to search for immunopeptides in the nervous system, and before long Candace found those too. Her work confirmed Blalock's discovery and took it a step further, pinpointing the chemical mechanism that enables a network-based exchange.

Peptides, Candace realized, were the body's messengers or "information molecules," circulating data that connect the brain with the endocrine, immune, and gastrointestinal systems in a constant feed-back loop. Neuronal activity did not occur only at the synapse level, as previously believed; she found that peptides flow throughout the body, finding "nerve hookups" with target receptors in regions distant from the brain in the organs, glands, bone marrow, lymph nodes, and nerve ganglia lining the spine.

These results had profound implications—namely, that the body influences the brain, and the brain influences the body. What we experience as a feeling or mood is the result of neuropeptide ligands, the process by which a neuronal circuit is stimulated simultaneously within the brain and body, which then spurs a behavior. *Rather than being a control center, the brain works in concert with other systems to generate thoughts and emotions—indeed, to shape our reality.*

Defying conventional wisdom, Candace believed that peptides and their receptors form the biochemical basis of emotion—that they are "molecules of emotion," linking the body's systems and organs into a pulsing, unified web that is constantly shifting and responding to inter-nal and external stimuli. "Peptides are the sheet music containing the notes, phrases, and rhythms that allow the orchestra—your body—to play as an integrated entity," she writes in *Molecules of Emotion*. "And the music that results is the tone or feeling that you experience subjec-tively as your emotions."

If this is the case, then our bodies aren't simply vehicles to carry around our heads, and the mind is distinct from the brain. Rather, the mind is mobile, as consciousness or intelligence is distributed along a vast, multidirectional highway of neuropeptides diffused throughout an organism at the molecular level. Following this logic, Candace main-tained that "the body is the subconscious mind." Body and mind are one.

Once again, Candace was navigating uncharted scientific territory. In asserting the mind-body link, she wasn't just pushing the bounds of her field; she was refuting the reigning paradigm established by René Descartes, the father of modern philosophy and science, that had defined Western medicine for more than three centuries. Cartesian dualism differentiated the soul or mind from the body, stipulating that the former is immaterial and thinking, while the latter is matter and unthinking. Based on this rationale, the pope had granted Descartes permission to dissect human bodies for study. They'd agreed that if the mind held the human's inherent sacredness, then once the soul had departed, the body was fair game for science and autopsy was not a desecration. Therefore, in suggesting the body's "innate intelligence," Candace was contesting the very basis of Western medicine, the foundation upon which modern scientific thought was built.

At the time, her views prompted eye rolls generally reserved for mysticism. The National Institutes of Health—nay, all of Western medicine—had been designed according to the Cartesian view, with a rigid hierarchy and silo-based funding structure that discouraged collaboration or information-sharing across sectors. Researchers who studied cancer, arthritis, diabetes, or pulmonary disease were pitted against each other as they jockeyed for grants. As a result, scientists worked narrowly in their bureaucratic stovepipes, breeding insularity and apathy, if not outright skepticism, regarding developments in other fields. Specialists clung white-knuckled to power and didn't take kindly to upstarts and outsiders questioning their hegemony or infringing on their turf—certainly not a woman, much less an incendiary woman like Candace. Though Candace would come to publish more than two hundred papers on peptides and was for a time the most cited scientist at the NIMH, it would be decades before her ideas were understood and accepted.

Despite the misgivings she withstood, linking body and mind seemed natural to Candace. Her corporeal and intellectual passions were frequently intertwined, and she sought partners who satisfied her yen for both. While, according to Agu, Rick Weber was "a rascal, the kind of guy you warn your daughters about," Candace found in Michael a thoughtful, reserved consort who was eager to follow her lead. Upon meeting, he'd explained that his curiosity about a possible mind-body link had been sparked by macrophages, the immune system's mobile scavenger cells that clean the blood and repair the body's tissue. He'd posited that for this to occur, macrophages must be communicating with other parts of the body. While Weber sought autonomy in his research, which he never would have achieved in Candace's shadow, Michael jumped at the chance to explore such notions under her auspices.

As their relationship turned increasingly romantic, Candace appreciated that Michael was open to adventures of all sorts, including those that pushed the boundaries of mainstream science. Where Agu seemed doctrinaire, Michael appeared bold and open to probing the practical applications of their mind-body work. He'd even explored alternative therapies such as bioenergetics, even though Wilhelm Reich, who'd inspired the practice, had been denigrated by the scientific community for controversial experiments with human sexual energy. In fact, when Michael returned from a weeklong bioenergetics workshop employing physical postures and sound to clear the body of trauma and stagnant energy, he was positively radiant. Just a year after her split from Agu, Candace found herself falling in love.

Though Rosenberg descendants loved with a tribal ferocity that absorbed people, including Agu, Mildred and her sister Lillian were wary of Michael. They saw him as a drain on Candace's resources who enjoyed basking in the glow of her prestige, and they questioned why someone with his strict Catholic upbringing would embrace an older divorcée. While Mildred accused Michael of riding her daughter's coattails, Lillian went further, asserting that he was "on the gravy train, a phony-baloney." "My mother couldn't stand him," says Candace's cousin Nancy Morris. "Mike had no social graces. He was sloppy and looked like he slept in his clothes. We always made fun of the fact that he would have to stand ten feet behind Candy. If she stopped short, he'd be up her ass."

Given Michael's comparative lack of responsibilities, the family also disliked that he diverted attention from Candace's kids. While Agu and Candace had been united in prioritizing their children's well-being, Michael seemed like a child himself, and with him Candace moved to recapture her youth. She'd spent her formative years either pregnant or in a lab, after all, while he'd been a wonky, studious teen with a limited social life. By the time they met, each sought excitement.

Mildred and the family grew alarmed when Candace left her kids waiting at daycare and regularly asked others to babysit so she could depart on weekend jaunts with her young lover. Candace and Michael would go skiing together, smoke a lot of weed, and trade on her status to land invitations to meetings in glamorous locations like Hawaii. "Michael was like, 'You get Maui Wowie on arrival? Let's do it!'" Deane says. "He wasn't saying, 'You're a mom. Don't you think you should be with your kids?' To him the kids were an inconvenience, but being with a younger man appealed to Candy's ego."

When Michael conjures their early days of dating, however, he portrays Candace as an assertive, alpha woman seducing a naive nerd seven years her junior. In his twenties, he was used to chasing women and had yet to be pursued; he'd never met a female as forward or cunning as Candace. Of course, Michael knew about her infant, but the first time he slept at Candace's home, he was shocked to encounter a little girl there in the morning. "Oh, that's my daughter, Vanessa," Candace said, shrugging. About two months later, Michael was thrown for a loop again when sixteen-year-old Evan emerged from the basement. "He says, 'Bye, Mom.' I'm like, 'How many more do you have hiding?'" Michael laughs. "[Candace] said she was divorced. Turns out she's not!"

Still, Michael was charmed by this impulsive eccentric who chafed against limits, a woman whose favorite saying was "If it's not fun, it's not worth doing!" Candace loved roller coasters and fast, flashy cars, owning first a Morris Minor, followed by a Hillman Minx, a Fiat, and a red convertible Spider—each of which she drove recklessly, regularly getting tickets and then ignoring them. "I had to fight her for control of the car," Michael says. "I'd say, 'Candace, you just blew through a stop sign!' and she'd say, 'I'll stop at the next one!'"

Michael grew entranced by Candace's boundless thrill-seeking. Once, when late for a flight, she lied to the gate agent, claiming to be a doctor en route to an urgent surgery. And when Bret "Hitman" Hart, the famous professional wrestler, hustled up behind her, she argued for him to board the flight too. In gratitude, Hart offered her tickets and backstage passes to his show later that night. At the arena, Candace clamored for attention in a crowd of mullet-haired lotharios and their half-naked girlfriends, and when sweaty Hulk Hogan exited the ring, she threw her arms around him. There was nothing this woman wouldn't do.

As their personal and professional collaboration deepened, Candace and Michael began attending a scientific conference each year in Colorado or Utah. Never one to let work get in the way of play, Candace would follow Olympic-level skiers down a slalom course even when her own skills were lacking. On one occasion, when competing against another female scientist, Candace pulled ahead and, cocky to the core, struck a pose for the videographer—before promptly falling flat on her face. When her clip played on repeat in the bar that night, Candace took it in stride, laughing, "Fuck, I had that bitch beat!"

Michael loved Candace's zest for life, and as they worked together closely in the lab, he observed her jazz musician's gift for improvisation, as she freely made connections, adapted, and shot from the hip. At speaking engagements, Candace was disorganized and constantly winging it, yet had a way of winning over crowds. She'd often drop her slides onstage, scoop them up in the wrong order, and put them in a projector upside down. Then, instead of being embarrassed, she would poke fun at her own clumsiness, dancing a jig while announcing, "Aaaand . . . the von Trapp family singers!" before dazzling audiences with her mind. In the dour world of science, Candace was a breath of fresh air. She made life fun, and Michael admired the bulldog tenacity that drove her—and him, by association—toward groundbreaking work.

Dubbing themselves "radical psychoimmunologists" (a term used pejoratively in a 1983 *Nature* editorial to caution against drawing premature conclusions based on their line of mind-body reasoning), Candace, Michael, and Rick Weber helped create not only the interdisciplinary field of psychoneuroimmunology (PNI) but also a new paradigm, a revolutionary, holistic way to understand and treat disease. Given their findings, it seemed not only possible but also prudent to address the mind and body together, linking physical symptoms with their emotional drivers.

Candace's peptide research had shown that what we experience as reality is constantly filtered through and regulated by our emotions, and much of these data goes unprocessed by the brain. As a measure of self-protection, so as not to become overwhelmed, the brain filters out a multitude of sensory information bombarding our bodies each day, absorbing only what it deems necessary for survival based on signals our receptors receive from peptides. Many emotions and traumas are therefore sidestepped by the brain and never rise to the level of consciousness; instead, they are stored at the body's cellular level, sometimes deep within the roots of our neuropeptide receptors. Accordingly, most of our actions are motivated by subconscious vicissitudes of emotions rather than a logically plotted road map dictated by the brain.

However, Candace observed that psychiatrists and psychologists generally treat the mind with no regard for its effects on the body. Likewise, physicians tend to the physical body without considering the impact of our thoughts and emotions. She insisted that, because they are linked, they must be assessed and addressed as an integrated whole.

As Michael had experienced when he tried bioenergetics, Candace contended that the mind could be healed through the body and vice versa. Given that receptors are malleable, she found that healers might achieve greater results by using the body as a "gateway to the brain," delving beneath the level of consciousness without the brain's participation to release stored negative emotions that she believed are the root cause of diseases such as cancer. "Your body is your subconscious mind," she argued, "and you can't heal it by talk alone."

Candace saw that unless we clear ourselves of stored traumas, we act largely on autopilot, with stressed-out central nervous systems that linger in fight-or-flight, our body's unconscious response to threats, even in the absence of clear and present danger. For instance, a child who has suffered emotional or sexual abuse often lacks the terms or context to grasp these offenses, and her brain may block or repress memories that are too painful to process. As an adult, she might continue to suffer symptoms of stress, insecurity, and anger, yet remain unaware of her core trauma.

Citing studies linking clinical depression with early childhood trauma and stress, Candace noted that when the body remains in adrenaline-fueled fight-or-flight, it begins to make the steroid cortisol. However, stress is compounded by steroid production, instigating a sequence in which stress creates more steroids and steroids, in turn, exacerbate stress, in a vicious cycle. If mind and body are one, cooperating in a fluid, integrated intelligence, then afflictions such as depression must be treated in a way that addresses the entire organism.

Contrary to most Western doctors at that time, and arguably today, Candace believed that our natural state is one of bliss—that we are meant to be in balance and that balance is best achieved by listening to the body's intrinsic wisdom. She hoped that her holistic perspective would complement the medical establishment's reductionist tendencies and that, by encouraging people to tune into their bodies' innate intelligence, she might engender a healthier population less reliant on expensive, high-tech medical intervention.

Candace's "bicoastal mind" bridged Eastern and Western medicine. As early as 1980, she'd begun researching and validating alternative therapies, as she and Agu, along with Larry Ng, a Western-trained Chinese psychiatrist and neurologist, showed that acupuncture stimulates the release of endorphins into the cerebrospinal fluid, thereby reducing pain. Her research also showed that the "emotional brain" wasn't limited to the amygdala, hippocampus, and hypothalamus, as previously believed; instead, it was spread throughout the body, particularly along the spinal cord, where two chains of nerve bundles channeled information-carrying peptides through a series of nodal points. Only later would Candace learn that these "hot spots" correspond to the chakras, or energy vortices, that ancient Hindu traditions credit with distributing life force. The forebrain, throat, heart, solar plexus, intestines, and genital/rectal areas are all vital to the autonomic nervous system, rich in neuropeptides and receptors.

Thus, Candace found herself second-guessing mainstream Western medicine, which identified energy in strictly cellular metabolic terms, and she began exploring Eastern notions of an animating vitality within all organisms. She came to believe that neuropeptides and their receptors were the scientific basis of what the Hindus called *prana* and the Chinese called *chi* (essential energy or life force), lending credence to the work of unconventional healers such as chiropractors, acupuncturists, and breathwork and energy practitioners who espouse somatic-emotional treatments to treat trauma stored at the cellular level.

Advocating what is now called integrative or functional medicine, or proactive steps to prolong and protect wellness long before the body grows ill, Candace began promoting natural solutions. When it came to drugs, she cautioned against overuse, exhorting that research should focus on understanding how our body's natural substances maximize our existing biology rather than constantly seeking solutions with exogenous medication.

However, Candace saw that instead of engaging in this more time-consuming work, many Western doctors advocated a quick fix in the form of drugs, particularly for mood disorders. After years of studying brain chemistry and neuropharmacology, she became highly critical of the medical establishment's "talk and dose" therapy, denouncing this strategy as "lots of talking and even more pills, which are supposed to make the unacceptable feelings go away." Many cases cannot be treated through the brain via psychoanalysis or antidepressants, and Candace grew frustrated that Western medicine offered no alternative.

Candace's evolving views had profound personal implications and further alienated her from her scientific family. In questioning traditional pharmacology, she was snubbing the field her mentors had conceived. Steve Brodie—Candace's scientific great-grandfather, who begot Nobel Prize–winning Julius Axelrod, who begot Sol Snyder— had launched the NIH's Laboratory of Chemical Pharmacology, investigating how chemicals affect and are affected by the human body, and facilitating the creation of synthetic drugs.

Historically, drugs had been sourced from nature; for thousands of years, healers had distilled the extract of medicinal plants to treat a variety of ailments. Organic chemistry subsequently made possible the manufacture of new drugs, but doctors and scientists were unable to evaluate their efficacy without knowing how they were metabolized by the body. Beginning in the 1940s, Brodie and his descendants unlocked this mystery, sparking a revolution in drug development that would yield untold profits for pharmaceutical companies. Was Candace now turning against them?

Though she lauded the healthcare advances that had sprung from the labs of her forebears, Candace came to believe that most mental health professionals were trigger-happy when it came to prescriptions. While her colleagues at the NIH worked hand in glove with pharmaceutical companies, prescribing antidepressants to mask the symptoms of a disorder, Candace believed they were failing to recognize and treat its underlying cause. Instead, she encouraged physicians to understand the ways in which stress and repressed emotions impact our physiology.

Candace also witnessed antidepressants and other drugs, particularly those given during childbirth, being prescribed without proper research into side effects that afflict not only the brain but also the body, creating a cascade of iatrogenic disorders, or physician-caused ailments resulting from a treatment intended to cure a patient. No one, certainly not pharmaceutical companies, had done adequate research to determine how these drugs affected the body's intricate feedback loop.

As an example, Candace reported that women on antipsychotic drugs often stop menstruating and experience the irritability, water retention, and weight gain consistent with premenstrual syndrome. Subsequently, to treat symptoms caused by the antipsychotic, doctors prescribe an antidepressant, which results in more and greater side effects, leading to further health problems and a permanent reliance on drugs.

Clearly, Candace's quest was personal, as she and her sister Wynne had been prescribed the precise drugs she was analyzing and coming to reject. Just as Candace was proving the mind-body connection and casting doubt on the value of psychopharmacology, Wynne was hospitalized for the second time and dosed with lithium, a mood stabilizer with acute side effects, including confusion, memory loss, and weight gain. Like Candace, Wynne felt numb on antidepressants; her creativity suffered and the extra pounds she carried pummeled her self-esteem, so she too ceased taking medication the moment she improved.

Wynne also functioned well for a time after going off the medications, but she inevitably relapsed. After falling deeply in love with a colleague at the Metropolitan Museum, she'd followed him to Boston and established a private restoration practice. But when that relationship fell apart in the early 1980s, so did Wynne. By then, Candace was in the throes of her romance with Michael and they'd planned a trip to Scotland, so Deane committed Wynne to McLean Hospital, where she spent two months convalescing. "That's where Michael was a very selfish man," Deane reflects. "He wasn't like, 'Let's postpone our trip. Your mother can't cope. Deane could use a hand.' Michael wanted to have fun."

Candace was also denying her bipolar disorder, however, and she didn't want a mirror raised by her sister. But once Wynne's symptoms were managed, she moved to Bethesda to be near family. Before settling into an apartment four floors above Mildred's at the Promenade Towers, a luxury cooperative, Wynne resided with Candace, who seemed best suited to manage her care.

Though Candace solicited advice from her network of mental health professionals, she often overrode it, and her tendency to commandeer increasingly caused disputes within the family. She denigrated the social worker Deane proposed because the woman lacked a PhD, and she pulled rank on Wynne's psychiatrists, who deferred to Candace as a world-class scientist. She advised against pharmaceuticals even as Wynne fell into deep depressions, and Deane feared that their middle sister might commit suicide without the help of drugs. "I was like, 'Stay out of it!'" Deane says. "But Candy took over even when advice wasn't wanted."

Candace was a revolutionary, and revolutionaries are seldom lauded in their time. Yet both her family and mental health colleagues came to see her as a mass of contradictions: a brilliant pharmacologist who despised the very drugs she'd helped create, and a woman who'd found the molecular basis of emotions but struggled to manage her own. When it came time for her next momentous discovery, Candace's greatest strengths—her singularity of purpose and blind faith in her own virtuosity—would prove to be her undoing.

CHAPTER SEVEN

THE PLAGUE

D ESPITE HER CHAOTIC, REBELLIOUS NATURE AND ICONOCLASTIC VIEWS, CAN-
dace had risen to become the tenured chief of brain biochemistry
at the NIMH. Michael's boss at the National Institute of Dental
Research, where he was based, had agreed to loan him to Candace's
lab, so in 1985 they were working side by side when she received a call
that thrust them straight into the center of the world's most exigent
health crisis: AIDS.

"Suddenly, fifty thousand people had AIDS, mostly homosexual
men. They were dying in the streets, and nobody knew why," Michael
recalls. "Americans didn't care about gay [men]. They were worried:
'Can it spread to us?' There was hysteria and alarm, people saying it
could spread through kissing or mosquito bites."

What appeared as sudden to some had, in fact, been an escalating
crisis for five years, as the United States government failed to act. Gay
men had been showing signs of exotic disease since 1980, and at the
Centers for Disease Control (CDC), scientists had been monitoring an
uptick in homosexual men suffering from symptoms like night sweats,

fatigue, diarrhea, and swollen lymph nodes, as well as opportunistic infections as diverse as psoriasis, Kaposi's sarcoma, pneumocystis carinii pneumonia, neuropathy, severe herpes and shingles, oral candidiasis (thrush), cryptococcal meningitis, toxoplasmosis, encephalitis, and Burkitt's lymphoma. Fungal infections that generally appeared in birds, sheep, cats, and deer were now being discovered in humans, as were cancers that attacked every area of the body.

To understand and halt the spread of a disease characterized by complex and mysterious infections and immune disorders required the collaboration of immunologists, epidemiologists, venereologists, toxicologists, virologists, and psychologists or sociologists who could identify patients' behavior patterns. Yet, as Candace had already experienced, such cooperation was hard to come by in science.

Knowledge and treatment of AIDS (acquired immunodeficiency syndrome) were primitive then, with false reports that its underlying virus could be killed with peroxide and Clorox. In 1983, the American Medical Association had caused a firestorm by issuing a press release suggesting that routine everyday contact might cause transmission. Tony Fauci, the ambitious young director of the National Institute of Allergy and Infectious Diseases (NIAID), was quoted as saying, "We are witnessing at the present time the evolution of a new disease process of unknown etiology with a mortality of at least 50 percent and possibly as high as 75 percent to 100 percent with a doubling of the number of patients afflicted every six months. . . . The finding of AIDS in infants and children who are household contacts of patients with AIDS or persons with risks for AIDS has enormous implications with regard to ultimate transmissibility of this syndrome. If routine close contact can spread the disease, AIDS takes on an entirely new dimension." Of course, these children had contracted AIDS in the womb or through blood transfusions, and Fauci blamed the media for taking his comments out of context. But by then the damage was done, with the public whipped into a frenzy of fear.

Making matters worse was a lack of adequate funding. As part of his presidential campaign, Ronald Reagan had promised to turn federal programs over to the states, which meant slashing budgets on federal health initiatives like the NIH. The administration refused to modify this policy, even in the face of a rapidly spreading epidemic that it claimed was its "number-one health priority." With subsidies and grant money cut, scientists saw no fame or prestige in curing "gay cancer" and focused their efforts on diseases more easily solved with limited resources, prompting censure that NIH stood for "Not Interested in Homosexuals."

This apathy stood in stark contrast to the nation's attacks on other health threats. For instance, in 1976, when a group of straight, white, middle-aged men who were members of the American Legion fell ill while attending a convention at a Philadelphia hotel, the government snapped into action. The CDC and Pennsylvania Health Department responded with unprecedented alacrity, determining within six months that the source of the outbreak was a rare bacterium that caused a pneumonia-like lung infection. The 182 afflicted (29 of whom died), who had been exposed by breathing infected water droplets from the hotel's air-conditioning unit, even had a malady named after them— Legionnaires' disease. Similarly, when cyanide was discovered in Tylenol capsules in the Chicago area in 1982, more than a hundred federal, state, and local agents mobilized immediately, coordinating with the CDC and the FDA. The government spent millions of dollars to learn that, most likely, a single lunatic had tampered with packages and killed seven people. No expense was too great when the lives of certain groups of Americans were at stake, and yet thousands of homosexuals were being hung out to dry.

As noted in *And the Band Played On*, Randy Shilts's defining account of the AIDS crisis's early years, in 1982 the NIH spent $36,100 per death on toxic shock syndrome, the etiology of which had already been identified, and $34,841 per death on Legionnaires' disease, compared to about $3,225 per AIDS death in 1981 and $8,991 in 1982. This meant that a gay man's life was only one-quarter as valuable as that of a member of the American Legion.

Evidently, the nation was plagued by another epidemic—prejudice—so no one was putting pressure on public officials. Meanwhile, religious fundamentalists had been working since 1977 to deny gay marriage and repeal homosexual rights, such as antidiscrimination laws and gays' ability to serve in the military, with Reverend Jerry Falwell and his Moral Majority leading the charge. "When you violate moral, health, and hygiene laws, you reap the whirlwind," Falwell preached. "You cannot shake your fist in God's face and get by with it." Denouncing gays' "perverted lifestyle," he claimed that AIDS was God's curse for repudiating "nature." Likewise, Jesse Helms, a senator from North Carolina, lobbied Congress to pass laws banning HIV-positive individuals from immigrating to the United States and slashing CDC funding for HIV prevention messaging toward gay men.

As a result, AIDS, which had an average incubation period of five and a half years, was permitted to spread unabated for the better part of a decade. Only when the virus had infected heterosexual populations through intravenous drug use and blood transfusions did the media sound the alarm and the government step in to help. By 1985, when the Department of Health and Human Services finally increased federal funding to fight the disease, the CDC estimated that hospital bills and lost wages and benefits for AIDS patients had already reached $5.6 billion and would soon rival the cost to society of cancer ($50 billion per year) and heart disease ($85 billion per year). Finally, with money pouring in, scientists were interested. "We had a global epidemic, a plague," Michael says, "and the NIH would take the lead."

Bob Gallo, the head of tumor cell biology at the National Cancer Institute, had catapulted to fame when he identified the human immunodeficiency virus (HIV) as the cause of AIDS, the condition that develops when HIV has significantly damaged the immune system. Estimating that one in seven people infected with HIV developed AIDS, Gallo called it "as efficient a virus as [he'd] ever seen." By then, three different research teams had discovered that HIV invades and infects cells by binding like an exogenous ligand to the T4 (later called CD4) receptor, which is found on lymphocytes, a form of white blood cells, in the immune system. The virus then depletes lymphocytes, making victims susceptible to opportunistic infections.

Gallo had found that the virus also infects brain cells, a breakthrough that explained the memory loss, depression, dementia, and neuropathy that clinicians were seeing in three-fourths of AIDS sufferers. This presented yet another obstacle in finding a cure: if the virus crosses the blood-brain barrier, then a treatment must too, but few medications were capable of doing so. Armed with this knowledge, Bill Farrar, an immunologist at the NCI who was familiar with Candace's papers on neuroimmune connections, phoned to ask whether the T4 receptor might be the entry point for AIDS in the brain. If so, perhaps this would explain "neuro-AIDS."

For Candace, this seemed an irresistible challenge. She knew that no one else was mapping immune receptors in the brain; most doctors and scientists still believed they didn't exist. Virologists were interested primarily in how viruses replicate, not how they enter cells in the first place. So Candace saw a unique path forward, a trail that she alone could blaze. She would use her cutting-edge knowledge of receptors to identify how the AIDS virus entered the cell and try to cut it off at the pass.

Candace mobilized her lab around this mission and quickly found that the T4 receptor showed patterns resembling those of established brain peptide receptors. She and Michael planned to present their data at the American College of Psychoneuropharmacology conference in Maui, and they arrived early to hike and camp in the Haleakala Crater, a dormant volcano. Michael had charted a course he mistakenly thought would be four miles from trailhead to summit, but instead he and Candace embarked upon an arduous eight-mile ascent with a vertical gain of four thousand feet. At the halfway mark, Candace turned a corner and saw a vivid rainbow illuminating the sky, which she took to be a sign that they were indeed on the right path.

"The rainbow, long a symbol to me of the promise of science to eventually reveal ultimate truths, now graced our way, beckoning us on," she writes in *Molecules of Emotion*. Their moment at the apex is memorialized in a photo that shows the couple resting on volcanic basalt against a backdrop of lofty peaks. Candace leans into Michael's chest, her head resting on his shoulder as he envelops her with his arm. "What Did I Get Myself Into?" she wrote on the picture. "14,000FT?!"

Once they'd descended into the crater, Candace felt her heart overflow with wonderment and her consciousness expand to perceive her own humble, yet crucial, place in the universe. This sense of peace and oneness followed her into the conference days later, and as she watched a slide show reflecting the agonies inflicted upon AIDS victims, she felt compelled to help alleviate their pain.

When it was Candace's turn to present, she was in a state of altered, disembodied consciousness as she displayed colorful slides of a monkey's brain and muttered aloud to the audience a thought that occurred to her for the first time right there. Repeating the logic of her opiate receptor experiment and the subsequent sprint to categorize endorphins, Candace proposed that if they could find the body's

natural ligand that binds to the T4 receptor, then they could manufacture a clone to block the virus from entering cells; essentially, they
could shut the door on the virus. A hush fell over the room as peers
absorbed her message. Candace was proposing a cure for AIDS.

Suddenly, as she uttered these words to the audience, Candace
heard a commanding, disembodied male voice urging her forward. The
approach she'd just suggested seemed so sensible that she felt compelled to heed the voice's instruction, and she would later write that
"whatever that voice was—hallucination, voice from God, my own
higher wisdom—I knew exactly what it was telling me to do!"

From Maui, Candace ordered $10,000 worth of peptides, then
raced back to her Maryland lab to begin the search. "She didn't agonize
over the decision or ask the group," Michael says. "She was all-in, all
the time." Querying a worldwide database that contained the molecular sequence of all known peptides, Candace and Michael spent a week
poring over printouts, laboring to find a structure that matched gp120,
as the aspect of HIV that fits into the receptor is called. Again, if she
could identify the T4's innate ligand, then she could create a mimetic
to block gp120 from entering the receptor. This way, the virus would
have nowhere to attach. As she and Michael homed in on the correct
sequence, he began to suspect that an octapeptide in the Epstein-Barr
virus used the same receptor, and he turned out to be right.

Candace also enlisted the help of Frank Ruscetti, a virologist at the
National Cancer Institute who had been studying HIV and was one
of few people in the world who could expertly isolate and grow human
viruses. When Candace arrived at his lab in Frederick, Maryland, to discuss partnering, he quickly recognized her vision and came to love her
mental pyrotechnics. "If there was a new and interesting problem, she
loved to tackle it," says Ruscetti, who had been the lab chief of leucocyte
biology before moving to the Biological Response Modifiers Program.

"Candace could generate novel ideas at the drop of a hat. She moved in and out of fields quite easily."

Candace told Ruscetti that she believed she and Michael had found the substance that mimicked the body's ligand to compete with HIV for receptors on brain and immune cells, and now she needed to know if it functioned as an antiviral. Would her peptides stop HIV from replicating in human cells? This was where Ruscetti came in, and it didn't take long to convince him to cooperate. "Candace could be very persuasive," he continues. "Years later, she would call me up and say, 'Frank, I have this idea!' I'd resist in the beginning because I had my own work to do, but after forty-five minutes of her saying how important it was, I always ended up doing her experiment."

Working with Bill Farrar, Ruscetti found with 80 to 90 percent effectiveness that, even in low concentrations, the peptides Candace had isolated also stopped the virus from breeding in human cells in test tubes. It seemed a slam dunk, and she felt as though Spirit had intervened. Candace's analytical brain was forced to acknowledge that every step of this process felt blessed, marked by some synchronistic blend of heightened intuition and extraordinary luck, and she sensed that she was being used as a channel by a benevolent higher power. How else to explain the sequence she and Michael had chosen and the ease with which they'd made this discovery?

The couple christened their compound "Peptide T" for threonine, the main amino acid in its molecular sequence, and moved to publish results they believed would lead to human trials. "It's amazingly satisfying to discover something new, something that's never been found before. If you can use it to help people, that's even better," Ruscetti says. "There are scientists who are most interested in making money off their discoveries. Candace wasn't like that. She just wanted to help people."

Others presumed Candace was helping herself, and straightaway she faced resistance. When a scientist in the NIH's intramural research program discovers or creates an invention that may be employed in the interest of public health, it is patented by the NIH's Office of Technology Transfer and licensed to the private sector for commercial use. If the commercial partner makes money as a result, a percentage of profits is funneled back to the NIH to fund further study. Inevitably, the researcher then commands greater resources and respect internally, and sometimes she is lured away to work for the biotech or pharmaceutical company, which enables her to capitalize personally. If, as with the opiate receptor discovery, her innovation has political significance, she might even become a household name.

As a result, the race to find a cure for AIDS incited the NIH's best and brightest, as well as its biggest egos. These players were hungry for fame and fortune, and many resented Candace for her previous triumphs. "You have to remember how competitive it was. The NIH was the center of the action. There was Bob Gallo, Sam Broder, and Tony Fauci all vying for the Nobel," Michael says of the NCI's head of tumor cell biology, the NCI's clinical director, and the director of NIAID, respectively. "People were forming coalitions, fighting for power, money, and prestige."

The AIDS crisis had caused internecine rivalries that had been brewing for years at the NIH to flare, as strident leaders battled for control. Once AIDS was identified as an infectious disease, Tony Fauci had begun his own pioneering research into human immunoregulation, shedding light on the human immune response and the ways in which HIV decimates the immune system to pave the way for fatal infections. This scholarship, which would make him one of the most-cited researchers in the world, required funding, and Fauci wanted resources directed to NIAID. Bob Gallo, however, believed that the NCI should retain control, as he'd begun working on the virus first. Their agencies were deadlocked and not communicating.

Typically undeterred, Candace loved scrapping with these highfliers. Gallo was already renowned for identifying the human T-cell leukemia virus (HTLV), the first retrovirus known to cause a human cancer, a feat for which he'd won the Lasker Award in 1982. In 1983, a retrovirus related to HTLV, which Gallo called HTLV-II, was unearthed by another scientist in his lab, securing Gallo's prominence in the world of virology. Tony Fauci was also a rising star who'd been tapped to lead NIAID in 1984 at age forty-three, making him the youngest person ever to hold the top job. Candace had known Fauci since they'd shared an award for standout federal servants under forty in 1978, and she believed him to be shrewd but fair. So, just as she'd done with opiate receptor research, Candace dove headfirst into the NIH's most belligerent scrum.

Though Candace was no stranger to conflict, the malice with which her opponents assailed Peptide T would come to shock her. In December 1986, when her paper was reviewed and published in the prestigious journal *Proceedings of the National Academy of Sciences*, she found herself in the spotlight again. Reporters at the *New York Times* and *Washington Post* heralded Peptide T as a port in the AIDS storm, and Tony Fauci was quoted in the *Washington Post* as saying, "For the first time, there is a synthesized protein which has been able to block the ability of the AIDS virus to get inside the target cell." In the same article, Sam Broder indicated that "this is a signal to pursue a new course for therapy." These men appeared, at least publicly, to support Candace and, with backing from her NIMH boss, Fred Goodwin, she was pushing toward a Phase I clinical trial to test for toxicity, or potential negative side effects, as early as the following year.

But then her rivals came out swinging. Immediately top virologists, immunologists, oncologists, and infectious disease specialists began disputing Candace's work, claiming that as an outsider in these fields, she couldn't possibly have uncovered something they'd missed; after all, if this were true, they'd have egg on their faces. Opponents denounced her not only within the halls of the NIH but also in the press, decrying her peptide research, spurning the mind-body link, and denigrating mental health as pseudoscience. "What business does a scientist at the Institute of *Mental* Health have treating a disease of the body?" they asked, conveniently ignoring that AIDS also infects the brain and discounting Candace's studies showing that the brain and body function together and may be healed together. No amount of scientific proof could shield Candace from this turf war with the "body boys."

Ruscetti dismisses Candace's detractors, writing off their criticism as conservative nonsense. Every important discovery is initially controversial, and it's common for competitors to claim it's in error. To make a leap and shift a paradigm, a scientist must prove predecessors wrong and replace their work. Predictably, those being eclipsed respond negatively and defensively, which prompts researchers to commiserate about the three stages of scientific recognition: "You're wrong," "You're an idiot," and "I knew it all along."

Ruscetti also observed Candace being singled out for ridicule because of her gender, as he'd seen his wife suffer similar bias. As a mouse virologist, Ruscetti's wife had chosen to remain at the NIH for the duration of her career because when she'd interviewed at a host of Ivy League universities in the 1980s and '90s, she saw no other women and knew she'd never win promotions or tenure. "A really creative person with innovative ideas is always looked down upon. If they happened to be female, they always got the worst end of the stick," Ruscetti says, emphasizing that the scientific community came down much harder on Candace than on him.

Sure, Candace had sharp elbows, but aggression in a woman is never appreciated. "Men can do it naturally and get away with it," he continues. "Women are supposed to know their place." Later, as an inscription in Ruscetti's copy of *Molecules of Emotion*, Candace scribed, "All the best to a great scientist with *total integrity*," which Ruscetti initially misread as "fatal integrity," prompting them to joke that the two were likely one and the same.

Though Candace got heated, she debated in a civilized, respectful way without personal jabs, unlike many colleagues who hit below the belt. Ruscetti recalls that, even in a milieu as polarized and hostile as the NIH was at that time, strikes on Candace were rabid. Instead of scholarly discourse, peers resorted to brutal trolling and mocking, assailing her character and appearance. "That's one thing I didn't like about our profession," Ruscetti says. "Reasonable people can disagree about data and it's not personal. You don't need to attack the individual. But people were particularly cruel to her."

Candace stayed positive in the face of rancor. On the wall of her office hung a postcard beseeching, "PLEASE—We have not as yet received your reply card for the Lasker Award Dinner, Tuesday, November 21, 1978," beside a poster that advised, "If you are getting run out of town, get in front of the crowd and make it look like a parade." The latter became Candace's motto for life. "It shows you that no matter what baloney you get in life, keep your eyes on what's important," Ruscetti says. "Your sense of self has to come first in a profession that depends on recognition and credit. Candace was good at that."

Yet if Candace was capable of perfidy, then how could she decry this trait in others? If she had perpetrated a ruse against her Hopkins friend Anne Young akin to that enacted against Peptide T, but cried foul only when the tables were turned, is it any wonder she lacked allies in her time of need? Regardless, Ruscetti says the system was rigged, and he speculates that biased colleagues circulated gossip and planted negative stories in the press to squash Candace and further their own gain. "There are a lot of bad actors in science," he laments. "What's that quote? 'Education doesn't change a man's character; it allows him to express it better.'"

Candace's adversaries had personal reasons for diminishing her work—namely, that they were developing their own treatments for AIDS and wanted to win. The National Cancer Institute prevailed after its leaders petitioned vehemently for azidothymidine (AZT), which had been originally created as a cancer drug in 1964 with funding from the NCI. When early results had been unremarkable, however, the NCI neglected to patent it. Twenty years later, when the NCI solicited companies for possible compounds to fight AIDS, the pharmaceutical company Burroughs Wellcome discovered that AZT was effective against retroviruses. The firm's lawyers shrewdly filed a patent before sending it back to the NCI as a candidate for testing. Subsequently, in early 1985, an NCI lab found that AZT stopped the AIDS virus from replicating in test tubes and Burroughs Wellcome funded a Phase II clinical trial of 282 patients.

Once early results showed that AZT extended a patient's life, the trial was cut short to fast-track FDA approval, which came on March 20, 1987. To understand the rarity of this occurrence, one must appreciate the exhaustive nature of the normal drug approval process. Generally, after a period of research and development during which only a small minority of compounds are deemed suitable for further analysis, a drug undergoes preclinical research. During preclinical research, scientists evaluate toxicity, or a drug's potential to cause harm at various doses, and results dictate whether the drug should be tested in humans. If so, scientists begin clinical research, or trials conducted according to established protocols in four phases.

Phase I, which lasts several months, involves twenty to a hundred volunteers who are either healthy or stricken with a particular disease and is intended to gauge safety and dosage. About 70 percent of those drugs move on to Phase II trials, which last up to two years and involve a few hundred people with the disease. Tests overseen in Phase II refine safety data and articulate questions to be answered in Phase III. About 33 percent of that set of drugs then moves to Phase III studies, which last up to four years and involve between three hundred and three thousand afflicted volunteers. These final trials, also called pivotal studies, define a drug's efficacy and, because of their breadth and duration, often bring to light longer-term and less common side effects. Less than 30 percent of drugs that have gone through Phase III trials are then approved by the FDA and move to the final phase, Phase IV, during which several thousand volunteers with a disease are monitored for safety after the drug has been released to the market.

The standard drug approval process can take the better part of a decade. However, facing pressure from the Reagan administration and the National Cancer Institute, the FDA approved AZT within twenty months, which is lightning speed in the world of drugs. Immediately, Burroughs Wellcome began charging exorbitant prices. At $10,000 per year (the equivalent of more than $25,000 today), AZT was rumored to be the most expensive prescription drug in history, and it arrived at a time when an estimated 35 percent of AIDS patients lacked health insurance or had policies that failed to cover drugs.

Researchers and clinicians initially attacked the virus with high doses of AZT (1,200 to 1,500 mg per day), instructing patients to take the drug every four hours, even throughout the night. Because these quantities resulted in severe side effects, including anemia, nausea, and diarrhea, many AIDS patients chose to wait as long as possible before resorting to the toxic drug. It would take years before researchers identified AZT's efficacy in lower doses when combined with other medications. In the meantime, AIDS patients were guinea pigs and Burroughs Wellcome swam in profits.

Despite public outcry for alternatives, other treatments seemed mired in red tape, stymied by squabbling bureaucrats who impeded each other's access to resources. Many in the healthcare community surmised that, in order to maintain both intellectual and market supremacy, the NCI and Burroughs Wellcome were purposely blocking therapies that emerged from other institutes or pharmaceutical companies. Journalists and AIDS activists began condemning the NIH for hindering drugs that were "Not Invented Here."

As the AIDS pandemic raged, Candace was embroiled in the fight of her career, trying to convince peers that her drug had merit. Everywhere she saw people tormented by a horrifying illness that stripped them of dignity before taking their lives, and she knew she could ease their suffering. Yet she felt cut off at the knees, sabotaged by an old boys' club that seemed intent on destroying her and her "child of the new paradigm," Peptide T.

Despite in vitro evidence of Peptide T's potential, with billions of dollars at stake and mounting public pressure, many were playing a zero-sum game. In a tactical blow, Tony Fauci commandeered $11 million of NIMH funds during a government budget meeting, strong-arming Candace's boss, Fred Goodwin, into retreat. Now forced to tighten his belt, Goodwin conceded that the NIMH would study the "softer side," or the social and behavioral aspects of AIDS, and cease competitive efforts to create drugs. Candace was left reeling from Fauci's land grab, and she suspected that it was rooted in backroom wheeling and dealing. Here she had a promising drug to treat HIV in the brain (and perhaps in the body as well), but she knew that without institutional support it would languish. So instead of courting favor and stroking egos—instead of being a nice girl who followed the rules—Candace once again went to the mat.

Moving to outsmart her "body boy" adversaries and gain traction for Peptide T, Candace sent a sample of her drug to Dr. Lennart Wetterberg, the head of the psychiatry department at the Karolinska Institute in Sweden. Unlike in the United States, where doctors must petition the FDA to administer an experimental drug on a compassionate basis after exhausting all existing treatments, Sweden allows its doctors to proceed at their own discretion. When Wetterberg gave Peptide T on a compassionate basis to four terminally ill men, their lymphocytes increased in number and brain scans (as measured by nuclear magnetic resonance) showed improvement of AIDS-related malfunction, with no harsh side effects. One patient who had a severe AIDS-related case of psoriasis saw his lesions disappear after four weeks of treatment; once he was taken off Peptide T, his psoriasis returned.

However, in January 1987, when Wetterberg's paper delineating these findings appeared in *The Lancet*, a top scientific journal, outcry erupted at the NIH. Bypassing NIH brass, Candace had taken her drug out of the country and aligned with a rival institution on the federal government's dime. Needless to say, NIH administrators were furious, and Fred Goodwin, who'd been Candace's staunch ally, was caught in the crossfire.

Candace's time at the NIH had been rife with impolitic exchanges, but by sending Peptide T to Sweden and attempting to circumvent the laws of her country and employer, she'd simply gone too far. "The evidence in her lab was extremely weak. Had she not sent it to Wetterberg, it would never have gone to human trials," says her collaborator Miles Herkenham. "If you know it's effective but don't know how, it's still not enough. But she was pushing it so hard—like Elizabeth Holmes of Theranos, massaging data to fit the story."

In March, the same month AZT was approved, Candace was invited to present her Peptide T results before a nineteen-member committee led by Fauci and composed of leading scientists from the government and top medical centers who were charged with deciding which AIDS drugs would proceed to clinical trials. In a letter to Dr. Frank Lilly of the President's Commission on the HIV Epidemic in December of that year, Candace reports that twenty minutes into her address she was interrupted by Dr. Martin Hirsch, the director of HIV/ AIDS programs at Massachusetts General Hospital, who also held positions at Harvard Medical School and the Harvard School of Public Health. Hirsch claimed that nine laboratories (which he refused to name) had tried and failed to replicate the results described in her *Proceedings of the National Academy of Sciences* paper. When Candace pressed for details, she was told that the committee would discuss the specifics only after she'd left the room. "What kind of smoke-filled old boy baloney tactics are going on here?" she seethed, claiming to have been "more angry than [I] had ever been in my entire professional life."

Next, Candace says that Dr. Cliff Lane, who worked at the NIAID under Fauci and had little or no exposure to her primary work, "volunteered a series of erroneous interpretations and subjective impressions to the Committee which needed to be vociferously corrected by Dr. Ruff, further lending to the carnival atmosphere of the proceedings." At that point Candace, Michael, Fred Goodwin, and Peter Bridge, who had been a co-investigator on the Peptide T trial, were forcibly escorted from the room.

"In our aggregate experience from Scientific Director to bench scientist, we had never encountered anything quite like this kind of treatment in all our professional lives," she writes. "I suddenly realized that the well had been inexplicably poisoned against Peptide T."

CHAPTER EIGHT

FAILURE TO REPLICATE

F ACTIONS WERE FIRMLY ROOTED BY MAY 31, 1987, WHEN THE THIRD INTERNA-
tional Conference on AIDS took place in Washington, D.C.,
cosponsored by the World Health Organization and the U.S.
Department of Health and Human Services. While the first two conferences had been smaller, laboratory affairs, this one was large and
highly publicized, in part because of the astonishing work of the sur-
geon general, Dr. C. Everett Koop.

Koop, whom the president had appointed based on his leadership
in the antiabortion movement, had stunned the Reagan administration
by spending the better part of a year interviewing scientists, policymakers, and gay leaders to fully grasp the scope of the AIDS epidemic.
His apolitical report presented AIDS as a public health crisis in need
of immediate attention. Against administration policy, it advocated
for AIDS education and confidential testing without the risk of discrimination against participants. President Reagan, who had yet to
give a single speech on the topic, finally felt the squeeze and agreed to
increase federal funding before the conference kickoff.

It was a heated moment in history, and Candace was already besieged. After other labs' "failure to replicate," she'd been systematically discredited in the media, as headlines regarding Peptide T shifted from "Research Suggests New AIDS Weapon" to "Scientists Uncertain About New Drug." At the May 1987 conference, Lennart Wetterberg was scheduled to speak about the results of his Karolinska study, but NIH officials intervened, demanding to see his materials and censoring his slides on Peptide T before they would allow him to take the stage. And, in a mortal swipe, Bill Haseltine, a professor at Boston's Dana-Farber Cancer Institute, Harvard Medical School, and the Harvard School of Public Health, stood up and echoed Martin Hirsch, declaring that he and his colleague Joseph Sodroski, as well as eight other labs, had performed Candace's experiment and failed to replicate her results. According to Haseltine, Peptide T showed no antiviral effects. "Peptide T does not work. Nothing. *Nada*," he told the *Boston Globe*, yet declined to discuss his data or methodologies with Candace and her team.

When she finally got access to these researchers' data, Candace learned that they had performed her experiment incorrectly. To repeat a test fairly, the concentrations of both the virus and drug must be consistent, but some of Candace's peers had increased the virus's concentration by a factor of 100,000 while keeping the concentration of Peptide T the same. As a result, these labs weren't repeating Candace's work; they were doing entirely different experiments. Moreover, their assays were relevant only in a test tube (in vitro), as the concentrations they used did not mirror how the drug interacts with the virus inside the human body (in vivo).

Once this information came to light, Candace's boss, Fred Goodwin, convened dozens of scientists on June 30 to foster dialogue and clarify the discrepancies in their findings. There, Elaine Kinney Thomas, a virologist at Oncogen, a Seattle-based biotech firm, reported that she'd repeated Candace's results, demonstrating that Peptide T blocked the AIDS virus at lower concentrations that are consistent with the virus's presence in the human body. Kinney Thomas had also found that Peptide T was more effective than AZT, as its therapeutic index, which measures antiviral potency against toxicity, was several orders of magnitude higher than that for AZT, which was still the only AIDS drug approved by the FDA. Regardless, the powers that be bowed to Harvard's Haseltine as he continued to bash Peptide T, forcing Larry Thompson, a staff writer for the *Washington Post*, to conclude in June 1987 that "the debate appears to be as much about the politics of science and the intense competition among groups within the AIDS research community as about science."

Rebuffed by her colleagues, Candace spent many days in a cage of despair. She couldn't stomach how rivals promoted toxic treatments while spurning Peptide T, a drug with zero side effects. Wasn't the point not only to extend life but also to improve it? And if Peptide T were snake oil, as her enemies claimed, then how to account for its anecdotal success?

Likening herself to virtuosi throughout the ages, Candace was adamant that eventually she would be proven right. She cited Galileo, who was tried and condemned by the Inquisition in 1633 for stating that the Sun is the center of the universe, and compared herself to Mozart in the film *Amadeus*. "The genius Mozart is given a review by his peer, the jealous musical expert Salieri, who pronounces his latest composition as having 'too many notes,'" she writes in her memoir. "It struck us that the problem with the Peptide T paper was that it also had too many notes, causing the 'experts' to find it too unfocused to comprehend."

Candace recalled the Hungarian doctor Ignaz Semmelweis, who was derided by peers in 1840s Vienna for suggesting that doctors should wash their hands before examining pregnant women. Semmelweis had observed that poor women treated by hospital midwives who scrubbed their hands were less susceptible to fever and infection than wealthier women in the care of doctors, who sauntered about covered in blood after sticking their hands into corpses. When Semmelweis and doctors on his ward began washing their hands in a solution of chlorinated lime, they found that less than 1 percent of their patients became infected. But without an understanding of germs, colleagues disparaged his ideas and subjected him to prolonged ridicule. Semmelweis eventually suffered a nervous breakdown and was committed to an asylum, and it would take forty years and the dawn of germ theory before hospitals prioritized cleanliness.

Candace also found a modern touchstone in Jesse Roth, a clinical director at the NIH in the 1980s who'd found insulin not only in the brain but also in single-cell organisms outside the human body. The medical establishment roundly rejected his discovery, averring that only a pancreas can make insulin, and Roth's papers were declined at every major journal until other researchers finally confirmed his results.

Citing cognitive bias, Candace consoled herself that radical leaps in science are never embraced, regardless of their origin, and scientists who've established a prevalent paradigm are disinclined to see their ideas overturned. Consequently, each novel or controversial idea is scrutinized, and often tarred and feathered, before becoming the status quo. This, Candace believed, would be the fate of Peptide T.

Over time, as knowledge of the AIDS virus increased, Candace, Michael, and Frank Ruscetti came to find additional reasons other labs couldn't repeat their results. The first involved the strain of virus used in experiments. In the mid-1980s, Ruscetti was one of a few researchers who exclusively used virus samples directly from patients because experiments with fresh blood modeled most closely the ways viruses infect the human body. Other colleagues, however, took an easier route, using lab-adapted virus strains that had been grown in test tubes. It would be ten years before scientists understood what a difference this makes.

HIV resembles the coronavirus, Ruscetti explains, because of its high mutation rate; the longer the virus exists within a patient, the more likely it is to change. As a result, in 1995, researchers ascertained that the scientists working with lab-adapted strains had been studying a variant of the disease that targets a different receptor. The strain Ruscetti employed straight from patients' blood samples targets the CCR5 receptor and is more clinically important because it causes infection first and is efficiently transmitted. After the virus mutates in the body, its variant targets the CD4 receptor. Sometimes the virus evolves to be dual-tropic, affecting both receptors. Peptide T blocks the CCR5 receptor but not the CD4 receptor, Ruscetti says, which explains why labs using the CD4 variant could not replicate Candace's results.

Perhaps this was an honest mistake, driven by ignorance rather than malice. Initially, Tony Fauci had been open-minded about Peptide T and, given the high stakes and urgency, had invited Michael to his lab during the holidays to repeat his experiment on the spot. "I had [Fauci's] guys looking over my shoulder every step of the way," Michael says. "His guy said it was maybe 50 percent effective, but it wasn't enough that Tony would put his name behind it. It's because they were using the lab-adapted strain."

To be fair, experiments are often hard to replicate and, in the 1980s, technology to measure HIV was crude. At the time, many scientists were adding high concentrations of the virus to expedite assays, and methods have since become more sensitive. "Lots of people try to reproduce results but end up doing it their own way. I would have people come to my lab and show them how it worked, but somehow it wouldn't get done right," Ruscetti says. "This happens all the time.

Four or five years ago, this guy took the leading thirty or thirty-five cancer papers published in a year and tried to reproduce them. He could
only reproduce one or two."

Similarly, in May 1987 Lennart Wetterberg of the Karolinska Institute, to whom Candace had sent Peptide T, reminded a reporter at the
New Scientist that when Candace first published her opiate receptor
findings in 1973, "many laboratories found it difficult to repeat that
work, although within one year, four laboratories confirmed that work.
That is now textbook knowledge." Wetterberg anticipated that within a
year Peptide T would also be vindicated.

That prediction never came true. At the NIH, "failure to replicate"
seemed a death blow, a final nail in the coffin for Peptide T. "Unfortunately, a small handful of very powerful scientists (government as
well as university scientists) wield such incredible power and influence
in the field of AIDS research that new avenues or approaches which
have not been developed [or] controlled by them are never pursued—
in fact, appear to be squelched," Candace wrote in her letter to the
President's Commission. "Moreover, government overseers (e.g., Dr.
Fauci), although well intentioned, are strongly motivated by a bureaucratic conservatism to make no mistakes, i.e., do nothing rather than
the wrong thing."

Less charitably, Michael and Ruscetti believe their rivals were
driven by greed. The men on Fauci's committee knew that the following year, the U.S. Public Health Service, which includes the NIH,
would allocate $1.6 billion to fight the AIDS virus, an increase of 78
percent over the previous year. By 1989, the Reagan administration
would increase that budget to $2.3 billion, more than the entire budget
of the National Cancer Institute, and about 20 percent would be spent
to develop new drugs. For the afflicted, AIDS was a scourge, but for
some scientists it was a gold mine.

The NCI's Bob Gallo, for one, seemed driven by a single goal. "Bob Gallo was into whatever would win him the Nobel Prize," says a colleague who has worked with him for forty years and, fearing retaliation, asks to remain anonymous. As this coworker notes, Gallo and his allies steamrolled anyone who impeded their path to glory, and Candace was one of many victims of their ruthless tactics.

Of course, Candace had heard rumors of Gallo's schemes, and when she approached Frank Ruscetti in 1985 to determine whether Peptide T had an antiviral effect, she also knew that just a few years earlier he'd been fired from Gallo's lab. Ruscetti had originally met Gallo at a hematology meeting in Atlanta in December 1974, where Ruscetti was searching for a job; his wife had already accepted a position at the NCI, and he'd hoped to join her there. Upon hearing Ruscetti's credentials, Gallo pitched a hard sell. "The first thing he said was, 'You want to come to a lab that's going to win the Nobel Prize,'" Ruscetti recounts. "That should have been a red flag." Gallo also claimed to Ruscetti, and ultimately to the world when he published in *Science*, that he had unearthed a new virus, HL23. However, in 1976, Gallo's reputation tanked when three different animal viruses were found to have contaminated his cell line. Perhaps Ruscetti could restore respectability to his lab.

Specifically, Gallo wanted Ruscetti to search for a human retrovirus that caused disease. As chronicled in "The AIDS Windfall," a damning 1988 exposé by Barry Werth in *New England Monthly*, Gallo's friend Dr. Max Essex, a Harvard virologist, had proposed early in the AIDS epidemic that its cause was a sexually transmitted virus. For years Essex had been studying feline leukemia, which is passed through saliva and sexual contact. Afflicted cats, he observed, were not in fact dying of leukemia, but rather from opportunistic infections that invaded once the animals' immune systems had collapsed. At the time, most scientists and clinicians decried the notion that cancers could be caught like infectious diseases, dismissing human tumor viruses as "human *rumor* viruses." But Essex and a handful of other virologists believed that if cats could transmit cancer, then humans could likely do the same. Whatever was causing AIDS certainly had the hallmarks of feline leukemia.

If Gallo's lab could prove the existence of a human cancer virus, then he would overturn assumptions, transform his field, and rehabilitate his image after the HL23 fiasco. According to Ruscetti, at least seven present or future Nobel Prize winners denigrated the notion that a virus caused cancer because they'd tried and failed to find one. And Gallo believed that if the virus existed, they would find it in myeloid cells that originate in the bone marrow. When Ruscetti hypothesized that T cells, a type of lymphocyte, might be a better place to look, Gallo insisted they'd yield nothing.

However, working with his clever postdoc Bernie Poiesz, Ruscetti found HTLV-I, the first human disease-causing retrovirus, which originated in T cells, just as he'd suspected. When Gallo learned of their success, he immediately swooped in for credit, winning the Lasker Award. "I should have won the Lasker Award for HTLV-I," Ruscetti says. "Candace's disagreement with Sol? That's mine with Gallo. She and I had a strange bond because we were both young and naive at one time."

Candace saw in Ruscetti a fellow underdog who shared her righteous indignation. She knew that after nabbing the Lasker, Gallo had refused to renew Ruscetti's contract, booting him from the lab in May 1982 after seven years of fruitful work. When he'd asked why, "Bob said, in a rare moment of honesty, 'You're getting too much credit,'" Ruscetti recounts. "Here was the guy who won the Lasker prize for my work, but he was essentially firing me because I was getting too much credit."

Ruscetti believes that Gallo then impeded him from being hired elsewhere at the NIH. After being unemployed for a year, he was finally welcomed by Joost Oppenheim, who ran the Biological Response Modifiers Program at the NCI branch in Frederick, Maryland. "Gallo had so much power that I went to everyone I knew at NIH, and nobody would hire me . . . but Joost did," Ruscetti says, crediting Oppenheim's courage to the fact that he'd escaped the Nazis in Holland. "He had been through so much adversity in his life that an asshole like Gallo wasn't going to threaten him."

Additionally, as Gallo's former colleague alludes, his assertion that he independently discovered HIV sparked an international incident that culminated in France's Pasteur Institute suing the National Cancer Institute in 1985. When Gallo had first studied AIDS, he'd been vexed by the knowledge that its cause was a retrovirus like HTLV-I, as he'd detected a retrovirus's reverse transcriptase enzyme in the lymphocytes of AIDS patients. The genetic code of retroviruses runs contrary to convention. Genetic information is normally stored in DNA and flows to RNA and then to proteins, which allow cells to function. Retroviruses, however, store genetic information in RNA, which needs the reverse transcriptase enzyme to copy RNA into DNA before infecting a host cell.

As a result, once Gallo's lab found evidence of reverse transcriptase, he suspected that whatever was causing AIDS was related to his leukemia virus. The problem was that while leukemia viruses cause white blood cells to replicate uncontrollably, the lymphocytes assailed by this virus were dying. It didn't add up. However, since "gay cancer" was an underfunded arena lacking potential for wealth and prestige, Gallo abandoned his search.

Meanwhile, in 1983 at the Pasteur Institute in Paris, Françoise Barré, a virologist who had once studied under Gallo at the NCI, also noted that the lymphocytes in her growth culture had perished, and she too suspected that AIDS was a retrovirus. Barré began running a radioactive test to detect the presence of reverse transcriptase every three days, before her lymphocytes had a chance to die off. When she saw enzyme levels peak in a short period of time, she realized what had baffled Gallo's lab. His researchers had waited too long, anticipating that infected lymphocytes would multiply as they did with HTLV. But whatever was causing AIDS didn't behave like HTLV. Barré was witnessing a new human retrovirus, and it was exceptionally lethal.

Discovering a new human retrovirus is a rare feat, and one that requires acknowledgment from the wider scientific community. As Barré and her lab chief, Luc Montagnier, prepared to publish a paper in *Science* on the retrovirus they would come to call LAV (lymphadenopathy-associated virus, because it had come from a lymph node), they sought Gallo's blessing. He was, after all, a patriarch of retrovirology, someone to whom scientists worldwide deferred. Bob Gallo had the power to validate their findings, so they shared their research and even sent him a lymph node from their Paris lab to study.

However, instead of acknowledging their work, Gallo circled his wagons, insisting that the French discovery was related to HTLV. Some researchers claim that he also badmouthed the French samples, alleging that they were contaminated, and that he warned the CDC against performing assays with LAV or collaborating with these "amateurs."

As reported extensively in both *And the Band Played On* and John Crewdson's *Science Fictions: A Scientific Mystery, a Massive Cover-Up, and the Dark Legacy of Robert Gallo*, Gallo was known to be territorial and vindictive. Once the Reagan administration opened its wallet to AIDS, he'd even drawn battle lines with agencies in his own country when he suspected they might surpass him in isolating the AIDS virus's root cause. When one of his mentees had the audacity to leave Gallo's lab to join the CDC, Gallo declined to share necessary reagents or anti-bodies, in order to throw sand in the gears of CDC experiments. Now that the French were closing in, Gallo was once again clawing for credit.

Candace and Michael were knee-deep in psychoneuroimmunology research then, watching from the sidelines as evidence mounted in support of the French LAV as the cause of AIDS. They'd heard that LAV belonged to the lentivirus family, primarily found in animals, and that Pasteur researchers had isolated LAV in the blood of hemophiliacs and detected antibodies in patients with swollen lymph nodes. The French had applied for a patent on LAV in 1983 and were working to develop a LAV antibody test for use in blood banks. Regardless, American science journals delayed publication of French studies and the Reagan administration failed to approve their patent, awaiting final judgment from Gallo.

Simultaneously, Frank Ruscetti, now in Joost Oppenheim's lab, was once again wrangling with his former boss. Unbeknownst to Gallo, NIAID's Tony Fauci had begun sending Ruscetti blood samples in hopes that he would identify the virus that caused AIDS. When Ruscetti was successful, making him the third person to isolate HIV, he wrote a paper and sent it to Fauci for review before submitting it to journals for publication. However, despite their flagrant enmity, Fauci and Gallo met every Wednesday for lunch, and Ruscetti claims that during one such tête-à-tête, Fauci showed Gallo his manuscript, and Gallo then tried to trick Ruscetti into sharing his work.

"Gallo was out for himself," Ruscetti says. "He calls me up and says, 'Frank, you have to send me that virus because the government can't be in the position of showing two viruses that cause the same disease. It'll look bad for the government, so please send me your virus and I will check it out.' I said, 'Bob, I'd rather flush it down the toilet than send it to you.' And that's what I did. I never published."

Because the NIH is a hotbed of gossip, Candace guessed that, to clinch victory for himself, Gallo would ensure that papers by Ruscetti and the French languished in obscurity while he moved to publish piles of scientific data about the retrovirus he was now calling HTLV-III, staking a claim by linking it by name to his earlier discoveries (HTLV-I and HTLV-II). Later, if LAV and his so-called HTLV-III were deemed to be the same, Gallo would have already cemented his reputation as its discoverer. In December 1983 he even informed the director of the NCI that he had found the virus that leads to AIDS, and the following April the NCI shocked the French by issuing a press release announcing triumph for the Americans, while ignoring LAV and the Pasteur Institute.

Ruscetti, who was awarded tenure and worked at the National Cancer Institute for nearly thirty-eight years until his retirement in 2013, told Candace that he sympathized with the French and felt ashamed of his government colleagues. While working in Gallo's lab, he'd even taught Luc Montagnier, who was then considered a friendly visitor, the technique to grow the T cells that Montagnier eventually used to isolate LAV. Who could have imagined that "this little-known Frenchman" would come to surpass Gallo and his fifty NCI researchers?

What's more, when Françoise Barré, whom Ruscetti had known from her early days at the NCI, was awaiting a response from Gallo about her initial findings, she'd called to ask whether the Pasteur team should dispatch more samples of their virus. Ruscetti had advised against it, cautioning that Gallo would steal her work. "I became a prophet," he says.

Some scientists, including members of the CDC, suspected that the French LAV and Gallo's HTLV-III might be the same virus, particularly after learning that Montagnier and Barré had shipped their lymph node sample to Gallo. In response, Gallo stonewalled attempts to perform genetic comparisons. However, in February 1985 at a press conference in New York, Luc Montagnier shared that the genetic sequencing performed by his team had shown LAV and HTLV-III to be identical. While Gallo claimed to have retrieved his sample from an American patient seventeen months after the LAV isolate was collected in France, Montagnier's sequencing proved that they were indeed from the same person, prompting a science writer from the *Philadelphia Inquirer* to ask, "Are you suggesting that Gallo swiped the virus from the French?"

Nevertheless, the Reagan administration, already beset for having dropped the ball on AIDS, put its full weight behind Gallo's narrative. A win for Gallo meant a win for the United States. While the French patent application had yet to be approved, precluding the Pasteur Institute from selling its blood test in the United States, Gallo's 1984 application for an HTLV-III antibody test was sanctioned forthwith. This enabled the National Cancer Institute to reap huge financial rewards on what was clearly a French discovery.

When the French sued for a share of the NCI's royalties, insiders knew they were also clamoring for recognition the United States had so arrogantly denied. Ultimately, to avoid public embarrassment, the case was settled out of court in 1987, when President Reagan and his French counterpart Jacques Chirac agreed to "compromise." Their governments would split royalties equally, and Gallo, Montagnier, and Barré were designated codiscoverers of a retrovirus renamed human immunodeficiency virus, so as not to show preference to either team. "Gallo was caught red-handed and nothing happened to him," Ruscetti says. "He got away with [it] because the U.S. government couldn't afford to shame him."

Empowered by President Reagan's support, Gallo and his Harvard cronies now sought to dominate the treatment of AIDS. As Barry Werth describes in "The AIDS Windfall," a 1980 U.S. Supreme Court ruling that expanded the definition of patentable discoveries had revolutionized biomedical research, and not necessarily for the better. Researchers no longer had to invent something to apply for patents; they needed only to have detected a commercially viable gene or molecule. Discoveries were suddenly characterized as "inventions" for which biomedical researchers could take credit and capitalize. Consequently, scientists who'd once shared research and materials freely were now incentivized to hide and hoard their most meaningful breakthroughs, creating a culture of secrecy and self-interest.

Bill Haseltine, the Harvard molecular geneticist boldly sounding the death knell for Peptide T, had jumped at this opportunity, founding Cambridge BioScience, a biotech company that was developing a rival treatment for AIDS. As Werth notes, Haseltine was a close friend of Gallo's, and he theorized that retroviruses were responsible for one-fourth of all human cancers. He'd procured the patent license for Gallo's HTLV-I and mapped its genetic sequence shortly after its discovery in 1981.

Meanwhile, Max Essex, who worked at the Harvard School of Public Health and had made the connection with feline leukemia, took an equity stake in Cambridge BioScience and served as an exclusive consultant. He'd discovered that HTLV-I also strikes the immune system and speculated that Gallo's retrovirus was responsible for AIDS. United by financial interest, these three men demolished their competition, including Candace and Peptide T.

Though Gallo's status as a federal government employee prohibited him from profiting directly from Haseltine's company, Barry Werth reports that Haseltine alluded to their strong alliance when he announced that his firm was "the group that played a key role in discovering the AIDS virus and it will have a lot to do with bringing you a cure." In September 1985, Haseltine's petition to the Senate

Appropriations Subcommittee for increased federal funding to fight AIDS no doubt helped Gallo. Notably, Haseltine was also elected to the Lasker Award jury in 1985, the year before Gallo, alongside Luc Montagnier and Cambridge BioScience partner Max Essex, won for their AIDS work. This made Gallo the only person in history to collect two Lasker Awards.

Haseltine, in turn, was appointed to the editorial boards of five scientific journals, as well as nine scientific committees, three of which made AIDS research funding decisions, between 1984 and 1987. With one hand washing the other, Cambridge BioScience soon had contracts with SmithKline Beckman and Institut Mérieux, a French vaccine producer, and by 1988 Haseltine's 350,000 shares were worth $4.7 million, while Essex's 150,000 shares were worth $2 million.

For Michael and Frank Ruscetti, this still burns. "Science and research institutions are in bed with pharma companies," says Ruscetti, whose work also triggered paradigm changes in hematology, including myeloid cell differentiation and stem cell regulation, the advance that initiated cord blood banking. "Since the National Cancer Institute and drug companies didn't find [Peptide T], they weren't interested in seeing it go forward. They want to only use materials they've discovered because they're patentable. They were in it for the money."

It wasn't until 1992 that the Department of Health and Human Services concluded in a sixty-two-page report that Gallo was guilty of scientific misconduct, making him the most senior researcher at the NIH to receive such rebuke. Officials stopped short of accusing Gallo of theft, however, allowing that his LAV mix-up could have been the result of accidental laboratory contamination. The following year, this verdict was overturned when Gallo showed that a third strain of the fast-mutating virus had contaminated first the French cultures and then the NCI's after the French sent him samples.

Not everyone was convinced, however. Despite Gallo's 1986 Lasker Award for his AIDS work, the international community later issued a ruling of its own. In 2008, the Nobel Prize for Physiology or Medicine was awarded to Luc Montagnier and Françoise Barré-Sinoussi of the Pasteur Institute, along with the discoverer of the human papillomavirus (HPV). Bob Gallo was conspicuously excluded. Though, as one colleague says, "he'll never win the Nobel because everyone knows he stole HIV from the French," Gallo was backed by the University of Maryland School of Medicine to cofound its Institute of Human Virology, where he has been director since 1996.

In the intervening years, many researchers came to find the Gallo-Haseltine-Essex triad suspect, and *New England Monthly* quotes Michael Lange, assistant head of infectious disease and epidemiology at St. Luke's Hospital in New York, as saying that three years were lost in AIDS drug development because of these men's stranglehold on the field. Bill Haseltine and his ilk should have been disqualified from assessing Peptide T, but with protectors in the federal government, no one would stop them from hip-checking contenders like Candace on their road to riches.

"Bill Haseltine's dick was bigger than Tony Fauci's," Michael says. "They had control over Tony, and Gallo wanted AZT because it came out of the Cancer Institute. So, we were screwed."

CHAPTER NINE

BLACK MARKET CANDY

A IDS REMAINED A DEATH SENTENCE, AND THE AFFLICTED GREW INCREASINGLY frantic. Because AZT was still the only FDA-approved drug, activists took to the streets chanting, "How many more have to die before you say they qualify?" to protest the glacial pace of drug testing and approval in the United States. As Randy Shilts reports in *And the Band Played On*, at the time less than 10 percent of AIDS patients in the United States received experimental drugs, and most sufferers were treated at later stages of infection, when their immune systems were already decimated. Drug studies take time, and patients knew that they'd be dead before these medications hit the market. "It was a free-for-all, a rodeo," Michael says, "with people searching the marketplace of ideas for anything that could help."

With no other options, AIDS sufferers and their allies self-organized, creating clandestine networks across the nation called "buyers clubs," which stayed abreast of the latest research, monitored experimental trials, and lobbied legislators for expedited approval and lower prices. Whenever possible, they illegally procured and disseminated the most compelling medications to AIDS patients well before they were FDA approved. Once drugs had been greenlit in other countries, American buyers clubs sent members abroad to purchase in quantity and sneak them across the border.

Buyers clubs first traded in drugs to treat the vast and varied symptoms of AIDS. Early favorites included ribavirin, an antiviral that combats respiratory syncytial virus (RSV, which leads to infections in the respiratory tract), hepatitis C, and some viral hemorrhagic fevers; and isoprinosine, which stimulates the immune system and addresses herpes simplex and genital warts. While these drugs were being evaluated in the United States, they had been approved for use in Mexico and could be purchased for less than 13 cents per tablet at pharmacies across the border.

Later, didanosine (ddI) became the underground drug of choice. This highly active antiretroviral therapy, which was developed at the National Cancer Institute to target HIV, became the second AIDS drug approved by the FDA—in October 1991, more than four years after AZT. Because scientists and doctors had not yet perfected combination therapies, many patients died before they could use their full supply, so friends and family donated the remaining stash to buyers clubs in hopes of extending someone else's life.

The FDA was aware of these illicit operations, but policymakers feared that shutting them down would backfire, and the government would be seen as depriving despondent victims of their Hail Mary pass. "People were sick, dying, and desperate. Our philosophy was that if something is nontoxic, if it won't hurt us, then why not try?" says Derek Hodel, who ran People with AIDS (PWA), the buyers club in New York, from 1988 to 1992. Hodel, who is now a senior program advisor at Physicians for Human Rights, says that while PWA, which was for a long time the largest buyers club in the country, strove to operate with integrity and transparency, complications inevitably arose.

"We weren't really qualified to say, 'This is nontoxic.' 'Nontoxic' is a totally relative term. Everything's nontoxic if you take it in the right doses, and the converse is also true. So, we really tried to be clear with people about what we knew and what we didn't know, and yet yield to individuals to make their own decisions," Hodel says.

Peptide T fell into a buyers club category called "what-the-hell drugs," most of which had an acceptable safety profile and strong efficacy data from overseas. Medications with demonstrated potential that had been sanctioned abroad included fluconazole (from Yugoslavia), an antifungal drug for thrush and yeast infections that is now commonly known by its brand name Diflucan; itraconazole (from Mexico), an antifungal that targets aspergillosis (fungal infection in the lungs), blastomycosis (Gilchrist's disease), and histoplasmosis (Darling's disease); azithromycin (now often called Z-Paks), an antibiotic used to treat bacterial infections, such as bronchitis, pneumonia, sexually transmitted diseases, and infections of the ears, lungs, sinuses, skin, throat, and reproductive organs; and clarithromycin, an antibiotic that addresses chest infections such as pneumonia, skin problems such as cellulitis, ear infections, and stomach ulcers. Each of these drugs was investigated and distributed by buyers clubs before receiving FDA approval and becoming part of standard care in the United States.

Select medications were also a focus of the Countdown 18 Months project, named for the average time from AIDS diagnosis to death for white males who were not intravenous drug users. Spearheaded by the Treatment and Data (T+D) Committee of AIDS Coalition to Unleash Power (ACT UP), the political action group formed in 1987 to push officials to respond to the AIDS crisis, the project's goal was to help patients survive the first generation of nucleoside-analogue antivirals in anticipation of better drugs to come.

"The antiviral treatments weren't coming online fast enough and weren't good enough yet to keep people from dying," says Garance Franke-Ruta, a member of ACT UP's T+D Committee, which was tasked with accelerating research for therapies. "It was the opposite of looking for a cure; it was people looking for a way to stay alive a few more months or even years so that if real treatments came along, they'd still be there to try them. And, barring that, to forestall blindness and suffocation and wasting for as long as possible." ACT UP also lobbied for interim prophylaxis guidelines, streamlined research procedures, and inquiries into less invasive and better diagnostic tests for opportunistic infections.

Though Peptide T had yet to present the clinical success of other "what-the-hell drugs," AIDS sufferers facing a quick, miserable death were willing to give it a shot. Consequently, Michael claims, Candace's sister Wynne took matters into her own hands. From her perch in the art world, Wynne had long known about the devastating illness striking gay friends. Now that she lived in Bethesda following her breakdown, she had a front-row seat to Candace's war on AIDS. Wynne began helping Candace with administrative work and accompanying her to the NIH, and then each night she'd hear Candace and Michael strategize about how to bring Peptide T to market. "Wynne was Candy's sidekick," Michael says, "thrust into this whole scene."

According to Michael, Wynne began cribbing Candace's formula for Peptide T and procuring dry peptide powder from Eng Tau, the owner of Peninsula Labs, a company based in Belmont, California, that supplied peptides to Candace's lab at the NIMH. Then she enlisted her chemist friend Larry Kwart to formulate an easily administered nasal spray that could be distributed by buyers clubs. "Maybe it started innocently, like Wynne's gay friends saying, 'Do you think you could help?' She probably thought, 'These are my friends, my people. Maybe

I can make a difference. People are dying and maybe I can save their lives,'" Michael speculates. "Wynne and Larry copycatted everything we did. They knew how we were making it for the clinical trial and made it the same way." From there, Wynne began reaching out to key AIDS activists in major cities, including Mark Harrington and Peter Staley, both of whom were prominent members of ACT UP, and John Perry Ryan, a leader of the Provincetown Positives, to launch an underground distribution network for Peptide T.

Rather than implicate himself and Candace in an illegal drug ring, which would be problematic even if the couple hadn't been federal government employees, Michael insists that Wynne and Larry Kwart acted alone. "They were taking a big risk. It was very cowboy," he says, avowing that when he and Candace discovered Wynne's far-reaching operation, they were shocked by her recklessness. "We said, 'Jesus Christ! We could be arrested. We could lose our jobs.' It would have been on page one of the *New York Times*. We would have gone to jail in handcuffs. We would have been destroyed!'"

It's hard to believe that Candace was kept in the dark, however, particularly when Michael portrays her as a puppetmaster in other areas of life. "Candace was the dominant member of that dyad, always rolling Wynne into her schemes," he recounts. "Wynne was more pliable. Candy always looked out for her and took care of her, and if Candy needed something, Wynne would jump in and shoulder the burden." Not to mention that Candace makes multiple mentions of her friend Dr. Jaw-Kang Chang and his wife, Eng Tau, in her memoir, praising them as her primary peptide suppliers who colluded, no questions asked, on a number of questionable ploys. Would Candace really have been excluded from their dialogue with her sister? Could Wynne have manufactured Peptide T on her own, or was she simply fronting for Candace?

In truth, Candace was running the show from day one, accumulating data from the burgeoning black market to combat her foes at the NIH. "How would Wynne start it up when she's not even a scientist or inside the NIH? She said, *'Let me get some secretly'*?" scoffs Candace's son Evan. "No, my mom brought it home. She was the leader. She had it in the fridge!" Candace's family attests that it was her idea to distribute Peptide T to AIDS activists—not to make money, but to bypass NIH rules at warp speed and gather anecdotal evidence for her drug. When Evan was living in San Francisco, she'd even arranged for him to meet a young man who had been taking black market Peptide T so that he could see firsthand the good her drug could do. "We walked along the Golden Gate Bridge area," he recalls. "He was the first person I knew who had AIDS, and he was dying and limping, but he felt better on Peptide T."

Candace had also given the drug to her children, and it had cured her daughter Vanessa's cold sore. She'd administered Peptide T to her uncle Henry Glasser, Lillian's husband, and it had cleared both his eczema and the brain fog caused by his myasthenia gravis, a chronic autoimmune, neuromuscular disease. And when her cousin David Glasser's nineteen-year-old son Jeffrey injured his spinal cord in a motorcycle accident, Candace overnighted a package of Peptide T to their home in Florida in hopes of controlling his inflammation.

"She sent us a powder and a liquid and told us how to mix it up as a nasal spray. She said to snort it like cocaine," says Peggy Glasser, David's wife. "I snuck it into the hospital. We had to be so secretive because Candy could go to jail because it wasn't FDA approved. The family knew, but none of the doctors or nurses knew." Jeffrey took a quick turn for the better, surprising doctors when both his facial bruising and the swelling in his spinal cord abated. The family credits Peptide T for the fact that Jeffrey is now paraplegic rather than quadriplegic.

Despite resistance from her adversaries at the NIH, Candace's tireless promotion worked. The first human trials to measure the cognitive benefits of Peptide T, or the drug's effect on neuro-AIDS, took place in 1988 at the University of Southern California–Los Angeles County Medical Center. They confirmed the Karolinska Institute's findings that Peptide T was nontoxic, with no side effects in humans, and patients experienced weight gain as well as improvement in brain and nerve function, reporting better memory, motor speed, mood, and energy. When the FDA subsequently approved a clinical trial at Boston's Fenway Community Health Center, an LGBTQ health, research, and advocacy organization, demand for Peptide T from buyers clubs skyrocketed.

Candace believed that since Peptide T had been proven nontoxic, she could do no harm by disseminating it. Additionally, because peptides occur naturally in the body and can be sold as supplements, in Candace's mind she needed FDA approval only if she were billing Peptide T as a treatment for disease. "She wasn't conning," Evan says. "She honestly believed Peptide T would help people."

Buyers clubs knew that Wynne's product was pure, being formulated by Candace at the NIH, whereas drugs that emerged from underground labs might be tainted. So in exchange for the sisters' help, AIDS activists funneled information about efficacy back to Wynne, who kept detailed records on her clients. Her files were teeming with success stories. A man who'd had agonizing neuropathy walked his daughter down the aisle. A taxi driver who couldn't remember directions was now back at work. A businessman had stopped wetting his bed at night. Word of Peptide T's effectiveness spread among buyers clubs, and before long Wynne was filling orders nationwide, influencing markets in New York, Boston, San Francisco, and Washington, D.C.

"Maybe it started in Manhattan with close friends, but by the end she had a big network with an upscale clientele—office people in the art and finance worlds, not heroin users on the street," Michael says. "You didn't need to drive your ass downtown to some street corner. As soon as your credit card cleared, Peptide T was at your doorstep."

During this time, Candace called her cousin Nancy Morris to ask if Wynne could stay at Morris's home on Long Island for a few months to oversee a Peptide T study that was happening in Manhattan. "She said Wynne was running the study! Her artistic sister with no science background was running a study? Give me a break!" Morris laughs. "I was busy with two young kids, so I didn't think too much about it." Surely, Candace feared getting caught operating a black market from her house in Maryland, but Morris's house in a quiet New York suburb formed the perfect cover.

While Wynne and Candace never spilled the details of their undertaking, Morris recalls that during the four months Wynne lived with her family, the house phone rang day and night with calls from tortured souls, screaming and crying for help. Wynne was constantly running to the post office to mail packages to supply buyers clubs, and at least once a week she'd borrow Morris's car to drive into Manhattan with a large bag whose contents she never explained. "Candace called her every night," Morris remembers. "Wynne did not do anything without her direction."

Inevitably, competing operations sprung up. "It got to be territorial. Martin Delaney, a powerful guy who was close to Tony Fauci, was running a buyers club in San Francisco," Michael says of the founder of Project Inform, an AIDS education and advocacy group that urged the FDA to fast-track treatments. "He shut Wynne out there, and Ron Woodroof shut her out of Dallas. She kept talking about this gangster guy pushing her out of the way, taking over the Dallas market." If this is true, then the *Dallas Buyers Club* script is inaccurate, as it describes how Woodroof, the film's lead character, smuggled Peptide T from Mexico into Texas to feed a black market for the drug. Yet Michael and Candace's youngest sister, Deane, contend that Woodroof was Wynne's client before he found a cheaper source of Peptide T in Mexico and edged her out of Dallas.

"It was Candace's drug, Wynne worked with activists to bring it through the underground, and I was doing their media stuff for the AIDS conference in D.C.," Deane recounts. At the time, Deane worked for the Massachusetts Department of Public Health in the Human Health Resource Office, which was focused on AIDS, and she used her Rolodex of powerful journalists to plant positive stories about Peptide T's initial trials. Though the Beebe sisters go uncredited, the publicity they generated for Peptide T, coupled with a lawsuit Woodroof filed against the FDA regarding a ban on the drug, eventually helped ease FDA regulations to expand access to experimental drugs for patients with debilitating diseases.

Candace knew that Wynne's distribution networks were useful politically in advancing the cause of Peptide T, so she and Michael also began welcoming AIDS activists into their home with the hope that they could convince NIH leaders to reconsider their stance on Peptide T. "Wynne built these coalitions. She knew the most important guys in each market and helped get them on our side," Michael says. "The gay guys wanted a seat at the table. They wanted treatment and, once they saw it was working, they agitated for Peptide T."

By then, AIDS sufferers had grown furious with apathetic legislators and were campaigning hard for results. As ACT UP leader Peter Staley recounts in his memoir *Never Silent*, activists pursued a two-pronged approach, negotiating with government officials and pharmaceutical executives when possible, while also staging public, and sometimes threatening, demonstrations meant to achieve policy goals. For instance, in October 1988, when the FDA refused to hasten the drug approval process, more than a thousand ACT UP representatives seized control of the agency's building in Rockville, Maryland, hanging a banner over the entrance that declared "Silence = Death." In April 1989, protestors locked themselves inside the headquarters of Burroughs Wellcome, AZT's manufacturer, to protest the drug's inflated cost. When their demands went unmet, they infiltrated the New York Stock Exchange in September, handcuffed themselves to a balustrade, and unfurled a banner urging "Sell Wellcome." Four days later, Burroughs Wellcome lowered the price of AZT by 20 percent.

When government officials dragged their heels or made empty promises, AIDS activists held them accountable. In May 1990, ACT UP stormed the NIH, sending two thousand demonstrators hurtling toward Building One, its main headquarters. Less than a year later, protestors who were livid over the Catholic church's anti-condom stance and invective toward gays demonstrated inside St. Patrick's Cathedral. ACT UP even managed to roll a giant condom over the roof of the house of homophobic North Carolina senator Jesse Helms, along with a note that blared: "A Condom to Stop Unsafe Politics. Helms Is Deadlier than a Virus."

Candace, Michael, and Wynne saw how activists made waves and moved to befriend them, hoping they would mobilize for Peptide T. These relationships proved mutually beneficial, Michael says, because after John Perry Ryan heard the case for Peptide T, "he jumped up, snapped into action, and barked orders to everybody." Michael credits the Provincetown Positives with paving the way for the clinical trial conducted at the Fenway Community Health Center, in which thirty-two HIV patients (thirty-one men and one woman) took the drug for six months. "We didn't have connections to Boston before, but Wynne was hooking these guys up with Peptide T and they saw it working," he says. "That's the reason that trial happened."

Dr. Kenneth Mayer, who oversaw the trial and is now cochair and medical research director at the Fenway Institute, recalls his interaction with Candace as "definitely one of these emblematic stories of the bad days of the AIDS epidemic," a time of rampant fear when science felt like a made-for-TV movie. Mayer was an infectious disease fellow at Brigham and Women's Hospital and studying molecular genetics at Harvard when he began working part-time at Fenway, running an evening clinic to treat sexually transmitted infections. At the time, Fenway tended to the area's large gay population, and Mayer had argued even before AIDS appeared that if doctors wanted to better serve their unique community, then they should engage in research as well.

The health center's board, however, resented Boston's academic research community for constantly requesting specimens for study, yet never reciprocating with results. For example, Fenway had provided stool samples from its patients to researchers at Tufts University who were concerned about intestinal parasites being reported in gay men, but Tufts failed to share findings that would have enabled Fenway's doctors to better treat patients. As a primary care center, Fenway objected to its patients being used as guinea pigs.

However, by 1981, when the first AIDS cases began to surface, Fenway leaders agreed that they were in a rare position to perform both research and clinical work. While Boston's teaching hospitals worked to palliate pneumocystis carinii pneumonia and other severe illnesses resulting from the AIDS virus, and Bob Gallo and Max Essex's labs labored to find its cause, Fenway was embedded in the trenches with the gay community.

"We would get calls at the switchboard saying, 'My boyfriend's sick. Does he have to stay in a separate room?' Or, 'My nephew is coming for

Thanksgiving. What do we do to protect ourselves?'" Mayer recounts. "I have some training in epidemiology, so we started to focus on what was transmitting this." Mayer saved blood specimens and, in collaboration with Gallo, revealed in late 1983 that 21 percent of his at-risk asymptomatic patients had antibodies to what Gallo was then calling HTLV-III (later termed HIV). This meant they'd been exposed and were poised to unknowingly infect others.

Generally, the federal government would not have partnered with a community health center for a clinical trial. But this initial research, which armed doctors with ways to optimize care, gave Fenway credibility for more sophisticated studies. Nonprofit organizations like the American Foundation for AIDS Research (amfAR), which was founded by Elizabeth Taylor and Dr. Mathilde Krim, a biomedical research scientist at the Sloan-Kettering Institute for Cancer Research, had been formed to fight government lethargy and were now funding community-based research projects with health centers such as Fenway as well. So Fenway was primed to collaborate when Candace arrived with a proposal.

Fenway's executive director during the AIDS crisis was Dale Orlando, who, as one board member notes, "never met a microphone she didn't like" and fearlessly faced down bureaucrats to enable the on-site delivery of experimental AIDS treatments. Orlando, who was passionate about behavioral and women's health, shared Candace's gusto and empathized with her plight as a female go-getter in a man's world. Candace's narrative—"that she's a brilliant neuroscientist impeccably trained at Hopkins who discovers this fundamental mechanism, and the traditional NIH establishment is freezing her out"—appealed to Orlando, who was also fighting an uphill battle, running a countercultural organization with rudimentary research infrastructure. "Here's this charismatic woman scientist at a time when there were certainly fewer women leading scientific enterprises," Mayer says. "Dale liked her, and Candace was fun and compelling about what Peptide T might be able to do."

By that time, Fenway had been funded by the CDC to do epidemiological studies, so Orlando believed that her center was equipped to perform a small clinical trial for a fellow female trailblazer. However, it soon became clear that this study would be a milestone for Fenway, requiring the organization to upgrade its facility and create an institutional review board to oversee the trial's protocol. If Peptide T were to be approved for use, then data had to be collected in a way that could withstand an FDA audit, which Fenway had never experienced.

When Orlando introduced Mayer to Candace, he was charmed but skeptical. Candace and Michael were, by then, plotting to leave the NIH to launch their own company and paying for the trial with $1.5 million in private company funds. To Mayer, this felt like a conflict of interest. However, knowing the players they were up against at Harvard and the NIH, he understood that the couple had no alternative. Fauci, Gallo, Essex, and Haseltine all had relationships that preceded AIDS, and it was natural that they'd lean on one another for guidance and results, rather than an upstart and outsider like Candace. "Max was a bona fide retrovirologist for years. This is a retrovirus, so the fact that Fauci might look to him for advice about retroviruses makes sense," Mayer reasons. "Candace is a neuroscientist who happened on this mechanism, so she's one or two steps removed and younger, so you can't separate out her age and her personality from the fact that she was a newbie to the field."

By this point, Tony Fauci had also recognized the necessity of engaging with AIDS activists, but his modus operandi was the inverse of Candace's. Fauci knew both his audience and his institution's constraints. He appreciated that ACT UP was led by bright people to whom he should listen, but he didn't make false promises or stray from his employer. "He didn't say, 'Tell me what to do,' or 'I want to use you to lobby Congress.' He was much more nuanced than that. It was more like, 'Tell me what's on your mind, so I can understand and try to be responsive'—which is a great way to be and also gives you deniability," Mayer says. "Remember, these were the Reagan-Bush years and he felt like he couldn't be too far out."

Unlike Candace, Fauci was effective working within the system. As detailed by Peter Staley in *Never Silent*, the NIAID chief promised activists that he would try to convince the FDA to speed the approval of ganciclovir, an experimental drug that prevented blindness caused by a viral infection in AIDS sufferers. Then, within five days, the *New York Times* reported that, in "an unusual move," the FDA was reevaluating its standards for the drug's approval and cited pressure from Fauci, who in turn credited ACT UP. "It wasn't lost on us that Fauci came off as a rescuing hero in the *Times* story," Staley writes. "Was he using us as much as we were trying to use him? Or were we simply on the same page by this point? . . . Regardless of motives, we decided to fully leverage our new relationship with the good doctor."

Months later, ACT UP presented Fauci with its recommended Parallel Track program, in which AIDS patients who'd been unable to enroll in experimental drugs' late-stage clinical trials could join a simultaneous observational trial. Soon after, Fauci pitched the concept in a *New York Times* article headlined "AIDS Researcher Seeks Wide Access to Drugs in Tests." "I call this a parallel-track approach to clinical trials," Fauci announced, taking credit.

As opposed to this suave and savvy diplomat, Candace was provocative and petulant, regularly trash-talking the NIH bureaucracy at Fenway's town meetings, even as Michael and their collaborator Peter Bridge were trying to work within the institution to gain support for

Peptide T. In many ways, Candace found a natural audience in Fenway's community forum, and she played to the crowd. "A lot of the Boston ACT UP people didn't have much use for the NIH, and here was this female scientist with a brilliant pedigree who's feeling totally shut out by the old boys' network there," Mayer remembers. "She engaged the community and was definitely highly regarded and highly irreverent."

Though Mayer felt sympathy for Candace, he also saw a manipulative quality in her interactions as she worked not only to help AIDS patients but also to serve her own purposes. "We had a great audience, great leverage. She's got nothing to lose and was looking for allies," Mayer says. "I never got the sense that this was about the money, but I think there was an intellectual narcissism—this idea that 'I've worked so hard to understand neuroscience, I've trained in the best labs, I'm the peer of people who've won the Nobel Prize, and now I've figured out this important fundamental biological mechanism that can really have a major impact on people's lives. So, why aren't people listening to me?'"

Though Candace mentioned to Mayer that she'd been distributing Peptide T underground, he avoided any direct knowledge for fear of implicating Fenway. Health centers are highly regulated, and it's rare for them to receive federal funding for research, so he needed to maintain distance from buyers clubs. "There were so many things Candace said that I took with a grain of salt, so I didn't know if that was organized or not," Mayer says. "The last thing I wanted was for Fenway to be associated with doing something illegal." Still, times were desperate and Peptide T had been deemed nontoxic, so he supported moving forward with the trial.

Looking back after decades, Mayer says that Fenway's study was hardly a textbook example of how to run a clinical trial and, like all

Phase I studies, it wasn't placebo-controlled. While Candace had been initially looking for a solution to neuro-AIDS, or cognitive impairment resulting from the virus, once Frank Ruscetti discovered that Peptide T had an antiviral effect, she became more interested in measuring the drug's effect on clinical progression. She wanted to position Peptide T as a cure for AIDS. However, the technology to measure viral loads had not yet been established and, because of HIV's long incubation period, it was nearly impossible to know how long a patient had been living with the disease. These variables made it hard, if not impossible, to measure clinical outcomes. As a result, much of the data collected over the course of the Fenway trial was subjective, and tension arose around how to interpret it.

Like Miles Herkenham, Mayer observed Candace's skewed perspective, as she saw what she wanted to see. "Candace made a lot of some of the in vitro lab findings that were not really validated as necessarily correlated with good clinical outcomes. There were one or two people who seemed to do well and she'd say, 'This is a real responder!' But we couldn't even know if there were subsets of responders," he says. "We'd have conversations where I'd say, 'Yeah, that's interesting and it may be really important, but you haven't really shown that yet.' We were very genial, but I think she was very disappointed that I didn't become more of an acolyte. I felt for her because she was really pushing and trying to move this forward as much as possible."

The majority of people who took Peptide T did report feeling better, however. While Candace and Michael assumed this meant that their drug was eradicating HIV, Mayer says that Peptide T may have been merely alleviating symptoms. It's possible that a small peptide crosses the blood-brain barrier to tickle a part of the brain that overrides discomfort, but Mayer recalls only a mild antidepressant effect, and the trial never unpacked these data.

Candace and Michael's new company had paid for the study, but the couple was stretched financially, "white-knuckling it." By the time the Fenway trial was complete, they still had neither a compassionate usage protocol nor a path toward FDA approval. And when trial participants who'd had a positive response learned that they could no longer receive Peptide T legally, they became enraged, accusing Candace and Mayer of unethical behavior. "Candace was very ambivalent about that because in her mind it validated how good the medication was," Mayer says. "She was thinking, 'What can I do? I don't have the wherewithal to do this alone.'"

Instead of proceeding solo, Candace again turned to activists. In September 1989 at the Institute of Medicine conference on surrogate markers, ACT UP chapters in New York and Boston, along with the Provincetown Positives, cited Tony Fauci's rejection of Peptide T as "proof of the lack of interest in constitutional symptoms and so-called 'soft' clinical markers as indicators of new drug efficacy," meaning that NIH officials disregarded AIDS patients' quality of life and well-being. The situation grew heated when Fauci, in turn, chastised Peptide T's developers for their "excessive zeal," and a member of the FDA's Center for Biologics Evaluation and Research accused Candace and Michael of subsidizing ACT UP to accelerate Peptide T's clinical evaluation.

A month later, based on what they believed to be promising results from the Fenway trial, these activist groups, plus ACT UP Provincetown and People with AIDS, joined ACT UP New York's Treatment and Data Committee in enumerating their complaints in a missive to Tony Fauci, copying President George Bush as well as a host of government officials and press representatives. "Peptide T has twice been submitted to the AIDS Clinical Drug Development Committee (ACDDC), and twice rejected," they wrote in a collective letter dated October 5,

1989, listing ten points that demonstrate "the bias and obstruction that have impeded Peptide T's development." "We believe that opponents of Peptide T's development were motivated by prior interests in competing therapies, and that these conflicts of interest have distorted the peer review process and its putative objectivity."

These activists maintained that Peptide T had been held to different standards of preclinical and clinical activity than other therapies the ACDDC had recommended. Most notably, they denigrated the committee's decision to push recombinant soluble CD4 (rsCD4), the treatment pursued by Bill Haseltine's Cambridge BioScience, into broad Phase II efficacy trials "despite the fact that rsCD4 has not produced any controlled data." The letter states that "rsCD4 has shown no clinical activity of any kind. In fact, the opposite has occurred. rsCD4 has an ephemeral half life in the blood (< 1 hour), and has shown no *in vivo* antiviral activity whatsoever. Nonetheless, plans for large Phase II trials are going full speed ahead."

Activists concluded by stating that "NIAID is riddled with conflicts of interest. ACDDC members are committed to competing antiviral therapies and are not motivated to approve one, developed like Peptide T outside the NIH system, which threatens the heavy academic and corporate investment in rsCD4. We demand that these questions of integrity and conflict of interest be answered."

AIDS activists were reading from Candace's playbook then, and they wanted to believe that Peptide T was the panacea she preached. "Candace was very convincing and was positive that Peptide T would end the AIDS crisis and HIV, ultimately, being an analogue to block HIV from entering the cells," says Anna Blume, who led ACT UP New York's Alternative and Holistic Treatment Committee in the early 1990s. "She called it a designer drug, designed to stop infection without toxicity. She had every reason to believe that Peptide T was promising, and she never badmouthed anything else. She was just a great advocate for what she created."

Blume became Candace and Wynne's primary contact and distributor on the underground in New York after the Treatment and Data group grew focused on AZT derivatives. For about eighteen months Blume was in regular contact with the sisters, lobbying the NIH on behalf of Peptide T while Candace supplied ACT UP constituents with free Peptide T. Of course, they all knew this was illegal, but obtaining permission to use an unapproved drug for compassionate use remained onerous and AIDS sufferers had no time to waste. "Candace and Wynne brought a whole box to my tiny apartment in Tribeca to deliver to friends," Blume says. "I remember bumping into someone who said, 'What are you up to?' and I thought, 'Am I a drug dealer now?' I had a strange feeling I was a drug pusher."

Blume didn't question where Candace was getting the drug, and they say that Candace never tried to extract money in return. To protect themselves, they were careful not to keep records, so they can't recall who took the drug or in what doses. If AIDS sufferers called PWA, representatives would give them Blume's number, and they would make the drop discreetly in local parks.

Blume came to understand why peers and activists were put off by Candace, however, and why ACT UP's T+D Committee members increasingly turned against her. When other scientists funneled drugs to the underground, they did so in a manner that was thoughtful and professional. But with Candace, everything was filtered through the lens of her personal narrative, and activists often felt that she was pressuring them to advocate for her. She also became obsessed with Bill Haseltine, constantly accusing him of treating her unfairly and undermining her.

"Because Candace took it so personally, doors did get shut. Perhaps if she'd handled it differently, there could have been more integrative dialogue," says Blume, who is now a professor of art history and museum professions at the Fashion Institute of Technology in New York. "There was this chip on her shoulder. You always felt that she was fighting, and it was hard to know if it was productive or not, that kind of mindset. . . . It was her script. It got a little tiresome, her ego and bravado, even for someone like myself, who thought what she was doing was wonderful and important."

Unfortunately, Blume, Franke-Ruta, and PWA's Derek Hodel report that, in their collective experience, Peptide T didn't work. Underground drugs for AIDS went in and out of fashion, Hodel says, and each one—including AL-721, a mixture of lipids extracted from egg yolks that was thought to reduce HIV's capacity to infect; dextran sulfate, an anticoagulant or lipid-lowering agent that was found to inhibit HIV-1 in vitro; and St. John's wort, which was believed to boost the immune system—had camps of supporters and detractors. "As soon as there was interest, there was money and there were promoters. We really tried to be careful about that," Hodel says. "There were tons of these things that came out where people said, 'I know the answer. It's cheap and it's nontoxic and it's going to fix everything.' We encountered it time and time again."

Though Hodel never met Candace personally, he remembers the hype around Peptide T and says that once PWA confirmed that it was nontoxic, representatives also began smuggling it into the United States from Copenhagen, which had a large gay population with easier access to experimental drugs. "My impression was that [Peptide T] didn't last long before people were like, 'Whatever, this is bogus,'" he continues. "Tons of things worked in the lab and turned out to be nothing. It doesn't matter how interesting it is in the lab, ultimately, if it doesn't work on people."

For their part, Blume concedes that many patients found Peptide T's intranasal delivery challenging and simultaneously were taking other drugs, which may have reacted adversely with Peptide T. Still, they say that none of the twenty to thirty people they knew who were taking Peptide T noted significant benefits. "The membership of ACT UP was sincerely and genuinely interested, and if the early trials had shown any benefit, we would have continued to support it," Blume says. "I wanted it to work, but Peptide T did not in any way stop the infection or end the disease. Of the people I knew taking it, to the person every single one of them died."

Candace was devastated by these reports. Why did Peptide T work under some conditions and fail under others? She knew that when Wynne and Larry Kwart operated alone, they were quick, overnight-ing Peptide T to AIDS sufferers who immediately ingested it. Yet once their operation scaled and buyers clubs were tasked with distribution, Peptide T was stored in refrigerators where the liquid aggregated, becoming thick and syrupy in nasal sprayers. Perhaps the drug was unstable, with efficacy decreasing with prolonged storage or changes in temperature. Solving this puzzle meant life or death—not only for AIDS patients but also for Candace's career.

CHAPTER TEN

SQUEAKY CLEAN

FTER OTHER LABS' "FAILURE TO REPLICATE," CANDACE HAD RETREATED TO her office, dejected that the positive results she was seeing from Wynne's clients weren't enough to garner support from the scientific establishment. In that dark and forlorn state, she got a call from a biotech lawyer that changed everything.

Bristol-Myers, the second-largest pharmaceutical company in the world, had performed Candace's experiment and validated her results and the results of Elaine Kinney Thomas at Oncogen, the Seattle-based biotech firm, who had defended Candace at Fred Goodwin's June 1987 meeting. This, in turn, had captured the interest of a billionaire investor and assorted venture capitalists. Might Candace be willing to join them, the lawyer asked, spearheading research and development to bring Peptide T, as well as other peptide drugs, to market?

It seemed a dream come true, not to mention a no-brainer given the backlash she'd faced at the NIH. In *Molecules of Emotion*, Candace presents this moment as an underdog's victory, a tale of tenacity rewarded. Drunk on a cocktail of "I-told-you-so," she appears enamored of her own pluck, asserting that she and Michael left the NIH willingly, on their own terms. "I was about to end my tenure and stroll away from the best deal in science that exists anywhere, the chance to work at the NIH," she writes. "But I didn't hesitate for a second. I was so determined to carry Peptide T forward that had my dead father appeared in a vision and pleaded with me to consider, I would have ignored his wishes." In August 1987, after supposedly submitting her resignation, Candace found a champagne-filled limo waiting to take her to the lawyer's office, where she signed a $6 million deal ($14 million today). Peptide Design was born.

Or so she says. Candace never let truth get in the way of a good story, and her brand of bravado makes for a riveting yarn. Gifted liars often tell the truth, but not the whole truth, and the *best* stories lie in the gaps. In Candace's case, this is a detail so tiny and seemingly irrelevant that it's easy to miss; under the terms of her new venture, she writes, Peptide T would be "in the bailiwick of a nonprofit medical research institution we called Integra."

Why would anyone place intellectual property into a nonprofit? From a business perspective it makes no sense. The expressed goal of a biotech firm funded by investors and a pharmaceutical company is to make money; executives secure a patent—or, in cases where the NIH owns the patent, then a license to develop it—with the aim of turning a profit. Yet Candace never explains why her nonprofit Integra Institute was central to this deal.

Michael credits a biotech lawyer who was married to an NIH colleague with finding the loophole that enabled the commercialization of Peptide T. Here was the problem they faced: Because Candace had developed Peptide T as an NIH employee, the NIH held the patent. Given that, as a federal agency, the NIH forbids its employees from using government labs and resources for personal gain, Candace and Michael found themselves in a pickle. They couldn't launch their firm

without a patent license, and they couldn't get a license while continuing to work for the NIH. The couple also feared that NIH administrators who were irate over Candace's rogue conduct would try to prevent
them from monetizing Peptide T. In a worst-case scenario, Candace
and Michael would quit their jobs at the NIH and be denied the
license, leaving them high and dry.

According to Michael, the lawyer devised a plan that allowed them
to remain at the NIH while building their company Peptide Design on
the side. He'd discovered that NIH lawyers had been sloppy; they'd
filed a patent for Peptide T in the United States but had neglected to
secure foreign rights, so he instructed Candace and Michael to grab
the rights in Europe. This effectively rendered both patents useless
because when rights are split, ownership is unclear and a potential
for lawsuits repels potential investors. Thus NIH officials knew their
hands were tied.

"[Procuring European rights] got us a seat at the table," Michael
says. "Once they learned we had Bristol-Myers and the billionaire
backing us, they agreed to give us the license, as long as it went into
our nonprofit Integra." When the terms of their contract with investors
and Bristol-Myers had been defined, Integra would transfer ownership
of the license to Bristol-Myers, enabling the pharmaceutical giant and
investors to profit.

If Candace and Michael wanted to hedge their bets, keeping their
jobs until the construction of Peptide Design's $2 million, state-of-
the-art lab was complete, then they couldn't appear to be illegally commercializing a product while working for the federal government. "[Our
lawyer] said, 'You guys are controversial. You have to be squeaky clean.
If a nonprofit holds the license, you won't be seen as money-grubbing,'"
Michael recalls, admitting that while cultivating a veneer of altruism,
they had money on their minds. "Integra would pay us handsomely,

like the head of the Red Cross gets a million-dollar salary. And it would fund our laboratories and research and give us control of disbursements if we all got filthy rich."

As Candace and Michael worked with their investor, the Pittsburgh industrialist Henry Hillman, and his biotech fund to get Peptide Design up and running, the NIH permitted Candace to remain in her lab to complete the projects she'd been running with her postdocs. "The NIH wasn't paying us anymore," Michael says, "but Candace had enough clout that they let us stay—until she pissed more people off." According to Michael, NIH colleagues were jealous that Candace occupied a three-thousand-square-foot lab and a corner office on the fourth floor, even though she was no longer an employee. Moreover, Candace did little to hide that she was using federal government space to grow a commercial venture and run an underground drug ring. She regularly brought Wynne and Larry Kwart, whom she'd hired as employees of Integra Institute, into the office, and Larry often stayed late in the lab, mixing drugs for buyers clubs.

"In the end, we got thrown out. They said, 'It's come to our attention that you're using our office space to promote your drug,'" Michael recounts. "I never had a tenured position, but they wanted to throw me out because of my nepotistic relationship with Candace." Imagining the uproar if the press latched onto the tale of a top NIH scientist using government dollars to moonlight as a drug kingpin, NIH officials allowed Candace to keep her pension provided she stayed silent. To avoid public embarrassment, they just wanted her gone.

By the time Candace and Michael were booted from the NIH, Bristol-Myers had assumed control of Integra's global license and their new lab at Peptide Design was nearly complete. In contrast to the drab government labs Candace was leaving behind, this ten-thousand-square-foot "futuristic fantasy lab" (the one nonnegotiable in her contract) would be a cathedral to her work, built to her sleek 1980s specifications—vaulted skylights, luxury lighting, pink walls, blue steel columns, rows of purple lab benches, an octagonal conference room, and a huge neon "Peptide Design" sign Candace had commissioned from a local artist. All of this was meant to make an impression: after years of feeling underfoot at the NIH, Candace would have the last laugh.

But it wasn't an impression her investors appreciated; she'd spared no expense on decor that was inessential to their mission, and when her initial staff of twelve more than doubled in less than a year, even her lawyer complained that she was spending money faster than she could make it. Her backers were similarly displeased when she planned a lavish opening party on August 8, 1988 (8/8/88), insisting on this date for its symbolic repetition of the Chinese digit for prosperity, despite the fact that a board member and lawyer were forced to return from their summer vacation in Maine. Further ruffling feathers, Candace coaxed another board member to announce, "It's now eight seconds, eight minutes after eight on eight eight eighty-eight!" while cutting a large rainbow ribbon to begin the festivities. For these WASP men in suits, her "semimystical themes" hardly inspired confidence. Candace had again failed to read her audience.

What's more, once their business was up and running, Candace broke into the phone system and changed the firm's outgoing message. "This is the company's porn system," callers heard. "For masturbation, press one. For oral sex, press two. For bondage, press three." Two weeks later, Candace and Michael's conservative, blue-blooded investors flew into town for a crucial meeting, concerned that they'd been victims of a security breach. "You mean voice porn? That was me!" Candace squealed like a giddy schoolgirl. "She proudly owned it—like, 'Wasn't it funny?'" Michael says, still dumbfounded. "They were so relieved that they were willing to forgive, but she could have gotten us in trouble. The phone system was like a Rubik's Cube toy for her—'*What happens if I push this button?*' It's a theme that repeats throughout her life. When she surveyed the landscape for correct behavior, she just couldn't see it."

In a rare moment of humility, Candace copped to the diva conduct and professional witlessness that led Peptide Design to become "Peptide Demise" just fifteen months after the company's launch. "Michael and I suddenly found ourselves—two people who had been shielded from having to deal with funding or budgets throughout their professional careers—sitting near the top of a multimillion-dollar bioscience venture," she writes in her memoir. "We had never played in this arena, and we proceeded to make a lot of mistakes."

Biotech firms seek to maximize rewards and minimize risk by exploring various applications of any given compound. If Peptide T was effective against multiple diseases, then the company would stand to make a bundle even if other AIDS drugs prevailed in the marketplace. Alternatively, the company would be well positioned if Candace and Michael developed additional products from peptides. The idea was not to put all their eggs in one basket. So, after allocating $1.5 million to the Fenway trial, investors pressured the couple to diversify their efforts. However, instead of following instructions, Candace remained fixated on AIDS, and with proving Gallo and Haseltine wrong. When she spent hours courting AIDS activists and continuing to fight the NIH instead of doing her job, executives lost confidence in her ability to execute. Bristol-Myers pulled back from Peptide T research and development to support ddI, the AZT derivative licensed by the National Cancer Institute, and Candace's biotech investors promptly closed up shop.

Now that Candace and Michael lacked commercial partners, they were left with nothing. The couple had no jobs or income and was relegated to working on folding tables in their basement, with a faulty fax machine they balanced on a crate in the bathtub; in a poignant metaphor, it sent but didn't receive. "Once we'd lost the protection of Bristol-Myers, we were naked on the street, abandoned and left alone to fend for ourselves," Michael says. "It was a very dark time in our lives." Still, they had to concede that Candace's incendiary behavior, a symptom of her bipolar disorder, was a source of perpetual strife.

The winter of 1989 was dire, save a small spark of hope that came from the Fenway trial. Though its results were inconclusive, a group of participants saw improvements significant enough to petition for continued use. However, Bristol-Myers's name was still on the patent license and the company refused to relinquish it, even though executives had no plans to move forward. In protest, Candace and Michael enlisted the help of John Perry Ryan and the Provincetown Positives, who had benefitted from the Fenway trial and who threatened to demonstrate in Bristol-Myers's lobby—and by "demonstrate," they meant fill it with contaminated blood. To avoid further menace, Bristol-Myers eventually gave up the license, at which point the NIH agreed to restore it to Candace and Michael's nonprofit Integra Institute, provided the couple secured a financial backer to develop Peptide T in the public's interest. Given the flop of Peptide Design, NIH administrators never thought that would happen.

Candace, however, was forever pulling rabbits out of hats. At a Medicine of the Future conference she attended in Germany in 1990, she had the good fortune to meet Eckart Wintzen, an offbeat Dutch entrepreneur who'd founded BSO/Origin, a computer software and services firm, in 1973. An iconoclast known for his long hair, paisley vests, and sojourns to Indian ashrams, Wintzen had a flair for management. As his company had grown, he'd divided it regularly into small, entrepreneurial "cells" to engender "friendly competition among peers."

More than two decades later, when he sold BSO/Origin to Philips in 1996, the firm had sixty-five hundred employees in twenty-four countries with global revenues of more than $500 million.

Simultaneously, Wintzen had been focused on environmental and social investments, and based on Candace's compelling presentation in Germany, he seemed willing to take a gamble on Peptide T. Just as the NIH Office of Technology Transfer was about to repeal any chance at licensing rights, Wintzen swooped in, wiring money from his bank account in Holland and pledging his support to Candace. Wintzen to the rescue!

Candace and Michael had scarcely begun to celebrate when, in an unprecedented and seemingly retaliatory move, the NIH split their licensing rights with a small Canadian company. Ironically, the reason the NIH now held the worldwide patent was that Candace and Michael had agreed to combine their European rights with the NIH's American rights before transferring the license to Bristol-Myers. Now the NIH Office of Technology Transfer was using this same split-license ploy against them. A divided license ensured that no pharmaceutical company or venture capital firm would invest and that Candace and Michael would never get FDA approval, which is bestowed only after a large sponsor has paid millions to shepherd a drug through clinical trials.

Wintzen learned of Candace and Michael's acrimony with NIH officials only after the fact, and he could have rebuffed them for obscuring the truth. Instead, he gave Candace the benefit of the doubt, spending five years fighting the NIH and their Canadian competitors for an exclusive license to bring Peptide T to market. The license would now be owned by Wintzen's company, Advanced Peptides and Biotechnology Sciences—later known as Advanced Immuni T, Inc. (AITI)—which employed Candace and Michael.

While Wintzen negotiated with the NIH, the couple secured research professorships at Georgetown University School of Medicine and worked from Georgetown's labs to help offset the cost of a series of minor Peptide T studies that Wintzen was funding. This included a placebo-controlled trial of eighty-one HIV patients at three medical centers in Manhattan, designed to measure the drug's effects on neuropathy. After results proved negligible, Candace and Michael learned that participants had undermined the outcome by meeting secretly in the centers' cafeterias to pool their medications. Instead of some AIDS sufferers receiving Peptide T while others took placebos, their decision ensured that all had access to a lower dose of the drug. "They knew they'd probably be dead before we got results that gave them long-term access," Michael says. "They cheated us because they wanted to live."

Candace and Michael's last chance came in the form of a noteworthy trial that the National Institute of Mental Health had quite shockingly approved. Five years after NCI immunologist Bill Farrar made his fateful call to Candace asking whether AIDS might infect the brain through the T4 receptor, there was still no cure or treatment for the memory loss, depression, dementia, and neuropathy that tormented three-fourths of AIDS sufferers. So, relenting to adamant AIDS activists who'd agitated for Peptide T, NIMH officials convened ten university experts (six proposed by NIMH and four nominated by NIAID) to review data on the drug's effect on AIDS in the brain.

"Everyone at the NIH expected them to say it's a piece of shit, but the experts came back and said the data from [the Phase I trial at] USC looked good enough to do a clinical study," Michael says. "[NIH officials] were aghast, but it obligated them to allocate money from their budget." Though siloed within the NIMH, the trial was sponsored in collaboration with NIAID, which meant that Tony Fauci and his committee had oversight. Given their explosive history with Candace, leaders stipulated that she and Michael be kept at arm's length. The couple was by then NIH outsiders—or, as Michael says, "persona non grata, damaged goods."

Instead of accepting this edict, Candace became a gadfly, meddling in confidential affairs, demanding details of the trial from former NIMH colleagues, and soliciting scientists and doctors outside of the federal government to help promote Peptide T. She saw a potential ally in Dr. Jeff Galpin, a renowned clinician and researcher in infectious diseases and internal medicine whom she'd met when he was asked by the FDA and NIH to testify about a study whose results were being twisted to accuse gays of mental illness. Gays weren't crazy, Galpin had argued, but rather had the symptoms of neuro-AIDS that Peptide T was designed to treat. "We were fighting bigotry all over the place," he says. "We weren't just fighting AIDS. We were fighting for gay rights, against churches in the South saying God was giving it to gays as a punishment."

Galpin empathized with the AIDS patients he was treating, in part because he'd faced bias while pursuing his own path. He'd become an expert on epidemics after having nearly succumbed to polio in the 1950s, at age eight. During the late 1970s, Galpin had helped develop a precursor to the PCR test used for rapid diagnostics, joining a company that did the first gene therapy on HIV. He'd become widely recognized as an expert on HIV, working with patients through the Elizabeth Taylor AIDS Foundation and the Elizabeth Glaser Pediatric AIDS Foundation, and speaking publicly on radio and TV. Reporters from *48 Hours* had followed Galpin through his clinic and office, tracking four of his patients—including a homosexual, a hemophiliac, and a woman who'd received a blood transfusion and passed the virus on to her children—to show that HIV was an equal-opportunity disease.

Against a backdrop of mass hysteria, Galpin hoped that cooler heads would prevail, so he was hesitant when Candace requested his support. "Candace was a genius, an egotist, a good person, and a bad person. She wanted to do one study and have the world proclaim her a genius, the next thing to Jesus coming back," he says. "We all used to go to the meetings with Bob Gallo at the NIH, and she wouldn't stop talking. She thought she could bend scientific law—*I'm not going to wait for this! We've gotta get this out now because people are dying!*' She was so convinced that she was right."

But Galpin could see that Peptide T had merit. When one of his patients had a seizure that paralyzed half of the young man's body and a scan showed that his brain was being eaten by progressive multi-focal leukoencephalopathy (PML), an aggressive viral disease of the central nervous system that attacks cells that make myelin, Galpin petitioned the FDA to try Peptide T on a compassionate basis. "I said, 'This kid's gonna be dead in a week and there's nothing to lose,' so the FDA let me write it up as an emergency investigational new drug," he recounts, but is quick to clarify that although his patient had HIV, he was testing Peptide T's efficacy as a treatment for PML, which also occurs in patients with other diseases that lower immunity, such as multiple sclerosis.

Galpin's request was approved, and within two days of receiving an intravenous infusion of Peptide T, his patient emerged from a coma. "It seemed like a miracle," he says with a smile. "When he woke up, I said, 'What would you like?' He said, 'I'd love to go to the Dodgers' opening day.' I said, 'If you make it to April, you get my tickets.' He took my tickets two years in a row." Within two weeks, his patient was walking with a cane. Galpin continued treating him for two years with intravenous infusions of Peptide T, and then stopped when new treatments were developed to improve immunity. That man is still alive today.

Candace knew that favorable data from preliminary studies and uplifting anecdotal evidence like Galpin's had convinced the independent academic committee to greenlight a Phase II clinical trial for Peptide T. In 1990, the NIMH embarked upon an $11 million, five-year study to assess the drug's neurocognitive benefits. Conducted at three independent sites—the University of Southern California in Los Angeles (USC), the University of California in San Diego (UCSD), and the University of Miami—the trial was both placebo-controlled, meaning that some volunteers received Peptide T intranasally while others received a placebo, and double-blind, meaning that, to minimize the potential for bias, neither volunteers nor researchers knew whether participants were receiving Peptide T or the placebo until the trial's conclusion.

In the trial, 215 participants who had been screened for cognitive impairment were randomly assigned to receive either Peptide T or the placebo for six months. At the end of this double-blind phase, all participants were offered the option to receive Peptide T for an additional six months. During the trial, investigators at each site administered a series of tests to gauge Peptide T's impact on participants' cognitive impairment, including struggles with memory, attention, language, problem-solving, spatial ability, and visual-motor coordination. Once tests were complete, in a compassionate gesture, the study granted participants an additional option to continue taking Peptide T until investigators had completed their analyses of the drug's value.

In many ways, this trial seemed doomed from the start. The first problem was that Ellen Stover, a psychology PhD assigned to the Office of Behavioral and Social Sciences Research at the NIMH, lacked expertise and experience running a drug trial and seemed biased against Peptide T. "Ellen was very difficult to work with and she made the trial much more difficult than it needed to be," says Peter Heseltine, the USC professor of clinical medicine who had been principal investigator for the Phase I trials and ran the USC Phase II trials. "Her opprobrium descended on all of us who were the investigators. It was more difficult than any other trial I've been involved in."

Obviously, Stover knew that Peptide T was controversial and that supporting the drug could be ruinous politically after its creators had been ousted from the NIH. She also knew that the study antagonized Tony Fauci, who wanted all AIDS research money funneled through NIAID, and influential members of his committee, particularly researchers from favored universities like Harvard. "I remember being told that a single case study at Harvard was worth ten at any institution on the West Coast," Heseltine says. "It's apocryphal, but not untrue."

Heseltine, who is now professor of clinical medicine, infectious diseases, at the University of California, Irvine, had helped design the clinical trial's cognitive function endpoints, which are events or outcomes measured objectively to judge whether the drug or treatment being studied is successful. This required endless debates with Stover about whether his endpoints were scientifically valid, in part because cognitive function testing was not her area of expertise.

"Ellen was so dismissive of the kind of science we were trying to bring forward," he says, noting that at the time, physicians dismissed psychiatry as subjective "fluff," presuming that patients' symptoms could not be assessed quantitatively like blood pressure. In response, Heseltine clarified that the tests his group had designed were not psychiatric tests that measured subjective well-being but rather tests of cognitive function designed to assess the brain's ability to recall and process information in areas such as visual and auditory memory, visual/spatial functioning, and psychomotor speed.

Cognitive function tests are hard to design because participants get better at them; they learn. So researchers need to find ways to measure the same skills in an increasingly challenging way. This task is tricky but not impossible, and Heseltine's group was skilled at administering cognitive function tests that were repeatable. "People just didn't want to accept it, in part because it was not invented at the NIH and it was talking about cognitive impairment, a problem about which most AIDS researchers didn't know very much," he says. "We developed tests to study it in a scientific way, quantitatively, but that wasn't widely accepted by the AIDS research community."

Additionally, Peptide T was being administered as a nasal spray and, according to Michael, Stover decided to cut shipping costs by increasing the drug's concentration. "A pharmaceutical company won't even change the wrapper on the bottle, much less change concentration of the drug," he says. "But she doubled the concentration so she could send half as many bottles!" Years later, Candace and Michael learned from a source at the NIH pharmacy that participants were told to store Peptide T in their refrigerators, but because Stover's committee-based approach proved endless, the drug sat on ice for two to three years before being tested, even though its shelf life was unconfirmed.

"Ellen did nothing to protect the drug. She never checked if it was stable," Michael continues. "She didn't want any Candace fans on her team or to be accused of bias, but we should have at least been asked about the formulation of the drug." Based on the buyers clubs' experience, Candace and Michael wanted their concerns about Peptide T's stability incorporated into the study's protocol, but they were never given the chance to opine.

Additionally, because Stover had doubled its concentration, under refrigeration Peptide T turned from a liquid into a gel, making it impossible to deliver as a nasal spray. Participants were therefore instructed by the NIH pharmacy to remove a vial from the refrigerator a day prior to use, shake it vigorously, and warm it in their hands. Then, the NIH pharmacy said, the vial with its sprayer could be stored at room temperature for at least two weeks while in use.

Peter Bridge, who had been the NIMH project officer on the Phase I trial before Ellen Stover took over for Phase II, says that when he left the NIH to work first for Johnson & Johnson and then for Roche, he realized how badly the NIH was hampered in drug trials by inadequate resources. "Peptide T's formulation was expensive by our standards, but not by pharma standards. If we'd had fully staffed pharma activity, then it would have gone more smoothly," he says. "We did the best job we knew how to do, but looking back after experience at pharmaceutical companies, I realize it was not enough. We didn't have the personnel or expertise to carry this out properly."

Compounding this comedy (or rather, tragedy) of errors, because of flaws in the study's protocols, administrators at some sites admitted patients who did not meet inclusion criteria for cognitive impairment, defined as "significant decline in cognitive function in comparison to their premorbid IQ." Said another way, Stover's trial allowed volunteers without substantial AIDS-related mental deficiencies to be included.

Researchers at the test sites knew that the study was fundamentally unsound, but they had no recourse once its protocols were established. According to J. Hampton Atkinson, who directed the trial's UCSD site, in a Phase II study such as this, his role as principal investigator was to oversee and conduct the study, recruiting participants, ensuring the safety of human research volunteers, and supervising the administration of assessments, data analysis, and fiscal management. He stresses that because the universities had signed contracts with the NIMH, they were not at liberty to change the trial's parameters.

"The investigators were not responsible for the scientific design of the research. Instead, the university (and I as the PI) entered into an agreement to carry out a scientific study—a research protocol—that was designed by the NIMH," says Atkinson, who is now professor-in-residence emeritus in the Department of Psychiatry at UCSD and was one of the founding codirectors of the HIV Neurobehavioral Research Center. "The everyday analogy is that the university sites in this multisite study were 'contractors' who agreed to follow a predetermined blueprint to construct a building."

The study was already under way when Atkinson's colleague Robert K. Heaton, who is now distinguished professor in the Department of Psychiatry at UCSD School of Medicine, joined the UCSD site. Heaton says that the trial's basic design called for initially using a brief neurocognitive screening battery to identify and enroll participants who were suspected of having neurocognitive impairment, and then administering a more comprehensive neurocognitive battery before and after the treatment period.

However, when Heaton arrived, he determined that the tests Stover had approved were ineffective, as a significant minority of participants did not show neurocognitive impairment on the comprehensive, baseline assessments. Heaton recommended that the team consider separately those who did, because the others arguably did not have the condition that Peptide T was designed to cure. At this point, Heaton was told that it was too late to change the approved study design, but that researchers could perform the analysis he recommended as secondary and include it in the final report, if warranted.

"In my opinion, ideally 'screeners' like this should be designed to avoid 'false positive' classifications of impairment, but when you find (after completing the comprehensive battery) that such false positives exist, you plan in advance that they no longer qualify," Heaton says. "But that is not what was done here."

Obviously, participants who were not impaired did not "improve" on Peptide T—because they were already mentally healthy! "Yes, I know this seems very 'wrong,'" Atkinson says. "I think the point is, however, that when a trial is designed, with predefined inclusion criteria and endpoints, by scientific convention the trial has to be conducted and reported based on this protocol (i.e., the result is reported based on a per-protocol analysis)."

Atkinson explains that this convention is designed to prevent investigators from cherry-picking results, for instance by first getting a negative result and then later identifying subgroups of participants who responded well and claiming benefits for a drug that don't exist for the majority. Years ago, the scientific community was alarmed that these types of subanalyses were used by pharmaceutical companies to hype new drugs; as a result, protocols are now followed strictly, even when studies have been poorly devised. "Unfortunately, in the case of Peptide T," Atkinson concludes, "the flawed study design (i.e., entry criterion) meant that a per-protocol analysis was doomed to failure."

Gauging the impact of a drug designed to improve cognition on a cohort of the unimpaired is like administering chemotherapy to a person who is cancer-free and testing for an uptick in health. There's simply no point. "Any drug company would have done the study just on people who showed a clinically significant level of impairment. If you can't remember the way to the grocery store, that's clinically significant," Michael says. "For people with no impairment, it's not important. Why would they even take it?"

Then, in another exceptional scorched-earth maneuver, in 1995 the NIH issued a press release declaring Peptide T useless, three years before the trials' results were fully analyzed and a white paper was published. This went entirely against convention, as press releases generally accompany the publication of a paper. During clinical trials, researchers collect data on an ongoing basis that are loaded into databases and examined for results. It is customary to determine top-line impressions, but these need to be audited and cross-checked for accuracy, and subsequently data are "cleaned" and surveyed for compliance in a process agreed upon at the onset of a study. However, instead of adhering to this approach, Ellen Stover issued a verdict on Peptide T before an evaluation was complete.

"The NIH white paper was disastrous. It essentially said the trials were a huge waste of time and money, which was disappointing for me," Heseltine laments. "I had an accountant telling me, 'I can't do mental math anymore,' and then after Peptide T saying, 'I can do it again. I've gotten my memory back!' These were encouraging things. I had to see [AIDS patients] on a daily basis, and ultimately watch many of them die. I thought we had found something to help, but our evidence was discounted."

As part of the NIMH study, USC also performed a brief clinical trial of Peptide T on patients who had cognitive dysfunction caused by chronic fatigue syndrome, which Heseltine says also showed profound initial results. However, because his group couldn't pinpoint a mechanism of action, outside evaluators attributed it to the placebo effect. But, according to Heseltine, when patients stopped Peptide T therapy, their symptoms returned immediately. "Maybe the AIDS research community felt that we were just trying it on everyone for everything and therefore it's got to be garbage," he says. "People said, 'Oh, you just found another way to fake the data or convince yourselves you were seeing something that's not really there.' It's the scientific process of disbelief. Usually that's helpful, but not if you want to get somewhere quickly."

In 1998, when comprehensive results were finally released, they showed that the primary analyses in Ellen Stover's final report were skewed and that Peptide T did, in fact, provide substantial benefits for patients in the bottom tier of cognitive functioning—exactly as investigators had observed. But by then, it was too late; Peptide T had been forever sullied when the NIH denounced it as worthless three years prior in the media.

Had the NIH press release indicated that Peptide T aided the impaired cohort, then the government would have been obliged to conduct further studies, which Ellen Stover wasn't keen to do. She was personally under fire by AIDS activists who demanded a verdict, but as Peter Heseltine points out, so was every research institution. At the time, he ran the largest AIDS clinic on the West Coast, which treated four thousand patients and was also a target for activists. "Everybody was appropriately frightened because they were pretty violent," he says. Heseltine personally witnessed protesters storm a pharmaceutical company and smash booths in its lobby, and his colleague was threatened by activists who knew where his children went to school and vowed to infect them with HIV because he wasn't working fast enough.

Similarly, when Stover's trials took longer than expected, activists began harassing her at her home, "pissing on doorsteps and demanding access. John Ryan got his teeth into Ellen Stover's ass and wouldn't let go," Michael says. "She didn't want to be bothered anymore. Saying [Peptide T] didn't work solved a lot of problems for Ellen and for the NIH. . . . The whole world was watching. This was going to be the definitive study, and they wanted to shut us down."

CHAPTER ELEVEN

SPIRIT OF TRUTH

B Y THE MID-1990S, CANDACE FELT DUMPED AND DISCARDED. INTRUDING ON THE NIMH study and condemning her former employer with AIDS activists had discredited her among scientific peers. Even colleagues who'd once marveled at her superpowered brain now distanced themselves, fearing tarnish by association. Candace and Michael had become pariahs in the world of science, banned from presenting at conferences.

"Candace was a very brilliant person. She saw molecules and was able to rotate them in her mind and mesh them in other molecules. You can do this with computers, but she could do this in her mind. She could see it," USC principal investigator Peter Heseltine says. "She did things in a very unorthodox way that damaged her reputation considerably, but I don't think she was a charlatan huckster."

Even with the best intentions, Candace lacked the skills and diplomacy to develop consensus, which is imperative in science. "Candace assumed that people who didn't understand her ideas were incredibly stupid, and that's not what people want to hear," he continues. "Science is about convincing your colleagues, and unfortunately some people don't want to believe for a variety of reasons—like people said the earth was flat. As my grandmother used to say, 'There are none so deaf as those who will not hear.'"

Steve Paul, Candace's administrator at the NIMH who'd helped recruit her from Sol Snyder's lab, says that despite Candace's credits and Frank Ruscetti's admirable reputation in virology, Peptide T was never viewed as solid science. He's surprised that they remained unable to execute a credible clinical trial and surmises that Candace struggled mightily with rejection, in part because she'd been showered with praise and attention so early in her career.

In his forty-five years as a professional scientist, Paul has learned almost never to declare categorical certainty. Some of the most important discoveries are discredited by others' failure to replicate results, often because they've conducted the experiment a different way, and theories that seem ludicrous sometimes turn out to be true. "Science is a self-correcting process with all the sundry issues related to human pursuit, like bias and politics," he says. "So, my view on Peptide T was always 'time will tell.'"

Paul, who after his time at the NIH spent seventeen years at Eli Lilly before launching a series of successful biotech companies, calls Candace a visionary and says that, in his experience, visionaries can be proven right overall, even when their initial reasoning is flawed. As an example, he cites Bob Heath, his early mentor at Tulane University, who believed in biological psychiatry, or that organic brain deficiencies cause mental illness. Notably, Heath felt that schizophrenia was a physical illness that could be treated by physical means. "Bob was discredited scientifically, but when you look at where the field has gone, particularly with regard to deep brain stimulation, you see he wasn't wrong," Paul says. "Bob was doing things sixty or seventy years ago that have now come back around."

With this in mind, Candace refused to give up. Despite insurmountable resistance, she and Michael continued to press for answers, and when tests to measure viral loads were developed, they begged to scan spinal fluid samples from the NIMH Phase II trial that were still being held in a freezer. Finally, after eight years, they got a call from a psychiatrist who'd been an investigator at one of the trial's sites. He asked to meet the couple "on the down-low" at an out-of-the-way bar.

"It was like Deep Throat. [He] sits down, leans in, and says, 'We tested your samples and it worked,'" Michael recounts, explaining that this psychiatrist had partnered with an NIH virologist to study the samples and discovered that Peptide T had an antiviral effect. When the couple asked what he planned to do, the psychiatrist backpedaled, claiming he was "gagged" by his NIH contract. However, Michael believes he was simply unwilling to expend political capital on their behalf. "[He] did this rebel thing by telling us," Michael says, "but because he got most of his funding from the NIH, in the end he was a pussy."

The psychiatrist's 2006 paper, published in the *Journal of Neuro-Virology*, states that "a DAPTA [a more stable version of Peptide T] treatment indicator variable was tested using generalized linear models on change in viral load. Peripheral load (combined plasma and serum) was significantly reduced in the DAPTA-treated group. No group differences in [cerebrospinal fluid] viral load were found. This retrospective study on a limited subgroup of the original trial sample indicated that DAPTA treatment may reduce peripheral viral load without concomitant CSF effects." In layperson's terms, this means that while investigators saw no benefits to subjects' brains, they echoed Frank Ruscetti's findings that Peptide T and its analogue meaningfully reduced viral load in patients' blood, thereby boosting their immune systems and reducing most symptoms typically associated with AIDS.

In the end, Peptide T was shown in some studies to improve neurocognitive impairment and in others to have an antiviral effect. Given this belated victory, one must again consider whether Candace's enemies were truly out to destroy her or whether she'd sabotaged herself. Both appear to be true. After the couple's banishment from the NIH, the quick collapse of Peptide Design had reinforced Candace's hothead reputation and shed further doubt on her credibility. A letter Candace wrote to Eckart Wintzen in August 2002 reveals that he too had lost faith and had been marginalizing her for some time.

"It is EXTREMELY IMPORTANT to me that you communicate with me as soon as possible," Candace implores, before explaining her desire to return to the lab to "resume an active research program" and "work on new cures." She then requests a meeting to discuss the possibility that she might begin a separate business venture focused on "non–peptide T technology," and offers Wintzen the opportunity to invest. "I have worked for you for twelve years and given every effort to make the PT project a success, and I will continue to support this with every fiber of my being," she writes. "I am not needed for you to go forward, I have little day to day role or purpose in running the Company . . . I need to move on and we need to resolve this."

Candace and Michael were rudderless, then. Despite their deal with Wintzen, who ultimately spent $25 million trying to bring Peptide T to market before finally closing AITI in 2004, the couple was facing bankruptcy, begging Candace's son Evan, who was thirty-eight, to move in to help pay bills on the new house they'd purchased while flying high on the windfall from Peptide Design. And in just a few years Candace had gained fifty pounds. Now even she was forced to rethink her approach.

"I'd incurred further establishment wrath by being an unquenchable spitfire when the NIH had refused to support trials for Peptide T, and I had earned more than a few enemies by insisting that I had the answer, the only solution that could cure the AIDS virus," she writes in her memoir. "It was a bitter pill to swallow, but I was forced to take a long, hard look at my behavior, my very unpolitic lack of respect and consideration for forces that seemed to so fiercely oppose me."

Over time Candace and Michael lost their allies in the gay community as well. AIDS activists had begun to align with Tony Fauci, who'd proven a valuable partner when he delivered results, including allowing activists access to key decision-making meetings within the NIH. His committee had already spurned Peptide T, and after the NIH press release in 1995, activists came to believe that the drug was a hoax. Some even maligned Candace as a swindler profiting from her lucrative side hustle.

These indictments trailed Candace and Michael, and five years later, in January 2003, Mark Harrington, who had broken with ACT UP to cofound Treatment Action Group, a nonprofit to expedite research, felt compelled to issue a point-by-point refutation of the couple's upcoming paper on the AIDS Treatment Activists Coalition (ATAC) listserv. Accusing Candace and Michael of wasting millions of taxpayer dollars on "nothing useful," Harrington condemns their efforts as "a really good example for everyone in ATAC of how NOT to do credible AIDS research, and how NOT to conduct studies (short-term, uncontrolled, unblinded, poorly characterized), and how NOT to analyse studies (selective use of data, shifting characterization of what's important, post hoc subset analysis, et al.)."

He writes that "[Candace's] statement that she hopes that 2003 is the year that 'peptide T gets the widespread access and testing it deserves' just shows her delusions—if she were a good scientist she would want the testing to come before the access, so that people would know whether the expense of yet another drug was worth it in terms of clinically and virologically meaningful clinical benefit. It's a bad paper, and it doesn't even deserve this much discussion." In a follow-on note, Harrington insists that "there's no news here, and certainly no breakthrough," and advises Candace and Michael that "it's time for you to abandon your own 'vivid dream,' and time to bring down the curtain on this distracting charade."

In 2013, Peter Staley of ACT UP told the *Washington Post* that Peptide T "never panned out. It's a useless therapy, and it never got approved, and nobody uses it today, but [*Dallas Buyers Club*] implies that it helped [Woodroof]." He revisits the issue in his 2022 memoir, criticizing early drafts of the film script as "a horror show for AIDS activism" and asserting that Woodroof supplied mostly bootleg ddC, a sister drug of AZT, rather than Peptide T, which he again decries as "a worthless drug that never got approved for anything."

By the early 2000s, the vast wave of AIDS-related deaths had ended thanks to antiretroviral drugs and triple combination therapies that halted the progression of HIV, and Peptide T had been surpassed by ostensibly better solutions. By continuing to pound the table for her drug, Candace lost authority as an objective scientist and instead was perceived as an arrogant, and possibly deluded, evangelist. In the eyes of the scientific community, her seminal work on the opiate receptor remained her crowning achievement.

Yet her opiate receptor discovery had also been co-opted and debased. Compounding Candace's humiliation over Peptide T was the rage she felt as pharmaceutical companies manufactured entirely new classes of drugs that treated the symptoms but seldom the root cause of disease. A war-weary Cassandra, she foretold what we now know to be true—Big Pharma had exploited her breakthrough. Instead of finding ways to liberate people from addiction, as she'd intended, executives churned out opioids that got people hooked.

At first pharmaceutical companies had worked furiously to create a nonaddictive painkiller fashioned after endorphins, reasoning that humans couldn't become dependent on the brain's own neurotransmitter. However, scientists were unable to synthesize a stable, endorphin-derived peptide that pierced the blood-brain barrier without producing symptoms of craving and withdrawal. Once it became clear that Big Pharma wouldn't make a mint by eliminating addiction, companies moved to create more potent analgesics.

The tragic irony of Candace's 1972 finding, touted in President Nixon's war on drugs as the first step to ending heroin addiction, is that it helped spawn a virulent epidemic of drug dependence that only worsened in subsequent decades. According to the Centers for Disease Control and Prevention, overdose deaths involving opioids (including prescription opioids, heroin, and synthetic opioids such as fentanyl) increased more than six times since 1999, and from 1999 to 2019 the nation lost nearly six hundred thousand people to overdoses of prescription and illegal opioids.

While overdose deaths from opioids hit a record high in 2020, driven by the enforced isolation and closure of treatment centers due to the coronavirus pandemic, Candace witnessed the first wave of these fatalities stemming from a surge of prescriptions in the 1990s, when pharmaceutical companies downplayed their drugs' potential for addiction to the medical community.

As chronicled in John Abramson's incisive book *Sickening: How Big Pharma Broke American Health Care and How We Can Repair It*, beginning in the early 1980s clinical research grew progressively privatized, aimed at enhancing financial return for shareholders. After President Reagan slashed federal government grants to universities and academic medical centers, researchers sought funding from pharmaceutical companies. The resulting financial ties created a conflict of interest, as Big Pharma influenced research studies to maximize their own profits.

By 1985, university scientists were benefitting personally from this influx of cash, as half of biotechnology research faculty members at top universities consulted to industry, while a quarter led commercial studies. This included Candace's colleagues. Sol Snyder had become a consultant to, director of, and chair of the advisory board of fledgling Nova Pharmaceuticals, which claimed to "utilize as its core business state-of-the-art neuroscience for the discovery of new drugs." When the company issued a $6 million stock offering in July 1983, Snyder benefitted. And after his mentor Julius Axelrod retired from the NIMH the following year, Snyder invited him to join Nova's scientific board as well.

By the mid-1990s, more than one-third of clinical faculty members at the nation's top fifty university hospitals were on Big Pharma's dole, administering chosen treatments to patients. And pharmaceutical companies had realized that they could avoid the bureaucracy and overhead of academic medical centers by creating in-house research and development units and hiring for-profit contract research organizations to conduct clinical trials. This enabled Big Pharma to control study design, own the data, and analyze and interpret it favorably for monetary gain.

Academic researchers, who were denied access to trials' complete underlying data, were hired to write reports based only on the limited subset of data they received from pharmaceutical companies. Predictably, this produced studies with slanted protocols and biased results. Ostensibly independent research reports functioned more as marketing brochures focused on profit rather than public health.

Remarkably, as Abramson reports in *Sickening*, this practice was concealed from the medical community. The creators of medical guidelines naturally assumed that research studies with the imprimatur of academic medical institutions were impartial. They had no idea that the manuscripts being submitted to medical journals for publication by academic authors were, in fact, corporate-sponsored, or that their original data had been withheld from peer reviewers and journal editors. Thus no one in the scientific community was in a position to judge whether studies were thorough or accurate. Pharmaceutical companies manipulated the narrative fed to unsuspecting doctors, who based treatment decisions on these "trusted" sources.

Candace knew that the most egregious example of this misuse of power was Purdue Pharma's promotion of its opioid OxyContin, which went on the market in 1996. In a widespread marketing campaign, Purdue fraudulently claimed that OxyContin was less powerful than morphine and could safely treat chronic pain; that the tablets' wax coating controlled the drug's release and slowed the body's absorption, thereby decreasing the risk of abuse and addiction; and that OxyContin was long-lasting enough to be taken only twice daily. None of these claims were true, but by 2001 they had propelled OxyContin to become the most heavily prescribed brand-name narcotic.

Unlike peer reviewers, the FDA has access to clinical trials' underlying data. Yet despite Purdue's dearth of evidence to support its declarations, the FDA approved a label avowing delayed absorption and decreased liability and made no efforts to monitor journal articles for veracity. Before long, it became clear that 21 to 29 percent of patients misuse opioids prescribed for chronic pain, and between 8 and 12 percent develop an opioid use disorder. An estimated 4 to 6 percent of those who misuse prescription opioids escalate to heroin, and about 80 percent of heroin addicts were initially prescribed opioids by physicians. Federal data estimate that the total economic burden of prescription opioid misuse alone in the United States is $78.5 billion a year, including the costs of healthcare, lost productivity, addiction treatment, and criminal justice involvement.

If the American scientific and medical establishment had lost faith in Candace, then she was justified in reciprocating. Now on the outside looking in, she felt bullied and betrayed, disgusted by a broken system that put outsized egos and corporate profits ahead of collective well-being. Facing the largest public health crisis of the twenty-first century, Candace was incensed that the Hippocratic oath—"first, do no harm"—would succumb to greed, and she was one of the few scientists courageous enough to protest. Like the creator of nuclear fission who came to hate the bomb, she saw her findings used for evil, with each new class of opioid lining corporate pockets while ravaging a population desperate for relief.

Candace's saving grace during these years was her mind-body work, which the powers that be had also panned but which was finally being validated. While her findings were dismissed during her tenure at the NIH, she now saw the Cartesian split of mind and body yield to a more holistic approach. Her alma mater, Johns Hopkins University School of Medicine, in a joint venture with academic and community hospitals and suburban healthcare and surgery centers, eventually espoused "complementary and alternative" medicine. And, in the early 1990s, the NIH created the Office of Alternative Medicine, which by 1998 had become the National Center for Complementary and Integrative Health, at last acknowledging and legitimizing treatments Candace had espoused for nearly two decades. Defining "complementary" treatments as those that use nutritional, physical, and/or psychological approaches and may have originated outside of conventional medicine, the NCCIH advocates the integration of these therapies alongside conventional Western medicine.

Candace's ideas were seeping into public consciousness, as stress, trauma, and anger came to be acknowledged as causes of disease. As the scientist who'd performed the initial mind-body studies, she was tapped for media interviews and increased her renown by appearing in Bill Moyers's groundbreaking 1993 book and PBS documentary series *Healing and the Mind*. She then cemented her narrative four years later with the publication of her memoir.

With a first printing of seventy-five thousand copies in September 1997, *Molecules of Emotion* became an instant bestseller. Deepak Chopra, an American-trained endocrinologist who brought ancient Ayurvedic wisdom to the West and achieved global acclaim as the "poet-prophet of alternative medicine," wrote the foreword. In 1990, before he'd become famous, Chopra had met Candace on a panel and invited her to the New England Memorial Hospital in Lancaster, Massachusetts, where he was chief of staff. There Candace had learned to meditate, and now he credited her with providing the scientific basis for his blockbuster career.

Candace's memoir tells a juicy tale of subterfuge, laying bare the dirty politics at Hopkins and the NIH and describing how, to cope with feelings of fury and desolation, she'd turned increasingly to spirituality. Interweaving her story with a primer on mind-body science, Candace recounts her journey from aspiring bench scientist to spiritual explorer, probing the prophetic nature of dreams and embracing the healing power of forgiveness as preached by Jesus. She explains that though she'd been raised as culturally Jewish, she'd begun attending services at a local church and singing in a choir, and she describes how she opened to the intuitive insights and psychosomatic treatments she now championed publicly.

Characterizing her creation of Peptide T as a divine epiphany following a moment of sacred communion with nature, Candace had come to view science as a mystical process, "like having God whisper in your ear . . . It's this inner voice that scientists must come to trust.

We must stop worshiping a dispassionate 'truth' and expecting the experts to lead us to it," she writes. "There's a higher intelligence, one that comes to us via our very molecules and results from our participation in a system far greater than the small, circumscribed one we call 'ego,' the world we receive from our five senses alone."

Candace believed that science was a vehicle for her own spiritual transformation and an expression of her God-given gifts. Through research, she sought the meaning of life in general, as well as her personal significance, and she'd begun to sense an interconnectedness, viewing the human body as a microcosm of the universe. Just as the body functions through coordinated, communicating systems, she reasoned, so the universe is an amalgam of integrated, inextricably linked components that form a greater, collective whole.

In modern times, spirituality or intuition is anathema in science, however; as Candace's NIH collaborator Miles Herkenham points out, the scientific method forbids it. So when Candace began using words like "God," "Spirit," and "soul" in her work, she knew she was uttering heresy. Yet she wasn't unique in chronicling mystical experiences or a heightened perception beyond the normal five senses, as history presents a long line of groundbreaking scientists, artists, musicians, and leaders who have attributed their inspiration to the hand of the divine.

In 1865, the German organic chemist August Kekulé claimed to have intuited the six-membered ring of carbon atoms of benzene in a dream in which he'd seen the ouroboros, an ancient Egyptian symbol later used in Greek alchemy and Gnosticism that shows a serpent devouring its own tail. Similarly, in 1869, Russian chemist Dmitri Mendeleev dreamed that he saw a chart classifying the fundamental sixty-three elements, giving birth to the periodic table. Nobel Prize–winning German psychobiologist Otto Loewi was also inspired by a dream to perform the first experiments on neurotransmitters and discover acetylcholine in the 1920s. Even Albert Einstein said, "I believe in intuition and inspiration . . . at times I feel certain I am right while not knowing the reason."

Most notably in the context of Candace's experiences, contemporary scientists conveniently ignore that René Descartes, a devout Catholic, reported having a series of three dreams in 1619 in which he was visited by the "Spirit of Truth." These dreams initially propelled him to consecrate himself to the Blessed Virgin Mary and vow to embark on a pilgrimage from Venice to Notre Dame de Lorette. But Descartes later came to view his visions as an exhortation to devote himself to scientific observation as his divinely chosen path. The irony of Descartes's famous declaration of reason, "I think, therefore I am," is that it was channeled from a transcendent place of open feeling. Central to this statement is a notion generally overlooked in modern times: Descartes's staunch belief in the existence of a God who has designed a logical, orderly universe for humans to discover.

As witnessed by the success of Candace's memoir, in merging science with spirituality she had tapped into Western society's deep need to address this duality. Scholarly advances in history, archaeology, and religious studies had shown many parts of both Old and New Testaments to be allegory rather than fact. Most educated people did not believe that God created the heavens and Earth in six days or that Eve had sprung from Adam's rib, much less tempted him with an apple that damned humanity with original sin. For millennia, wars had been fought on behalf of vengeful gods, and many questioned whether organized religion had been corrupted by vainglorious men consolidating power rather than living God's truth.

Still, the lessons of love, compassion, forgiveness, and acceptance inherent in religious texts applied, and people continued to seek a connection to forces greater than themselves. Increasingly, individuals were rejecting divisive, doctrinaire institutions and instead declaring themselves "spiritual," cultivating a personal relationship with their higher power. Candace, like Descartes before her, affirmed that divine devotion need not conflict with faith in science and technology. After all, both science and faith rely on the assumption that the universe consists of more than our five senses can perceive.

Following the publication of *Molecules of Emotion*, Candace referred to herself openly as a "recovering atheist" who'd abandoned the black suits of her "former life" in favor of colorful caftans. She catapulted to fame after appearing in the 2004 film *What the Bleep Do We Know?*, which investigated the link between consciousness and quantum physics. After it went viral, she blossomed as a New Age icon, hailed as the mother of the mind-body revolution and revered by stars such as Naomi Judd, who wrote the foreword to her second book, *Everything You Need to Know to Feel Go(o)d*. Candace became a sought-after speaker on the global mind-body circuit, joining luminaries like Deepak Chopra; Stan Grof, a driving force behind transpersonal or spiritual psychology; Willis Harman, a leader in the human potential movement; and Joan Borysenko, a bestselling author and cofounder of the Mind/Body Medical Institute.

"At mind-body events, she'd show up and there would be two thousand people in the audience," Michael says. "She'd do a few talks per month and people loved her because she gave scientific explanation for something they did." Consumer demand for alternative treatments was exploding as patients with access to information became less likely to trust implicitly the doctors they once saw as gods and instead seek solutions with fewer side effects. Mainstream, middle-class Americans were now practicing yoga and benefitting from acupuncturists, chiropractors, kinesiologists, and energy workers, but they didn't know why such treatments worked. Noting that "absence of proof is not proof of absence," Candace was happy to enlighten them.

Both in her memoir and onstage, Candace unraveled the psycho-neuroimmunology research she and Michael had begun two decades prior but which only recently had been accepted as scientific fact. She taught that the body was not static, as previously believed, but rather continued to make new neurons all the time, often straight from its bone marrow. As opposed to the head-first, top-down hierarchy that had dominated Western medicine, the brain functioned with the endocrine, immune, and gastrointestinal systems as a network with nodal points. Candace described how the neurons and ganglia that lie along the spinal cord and correspond to the chakras are rich in neuro-peptides and receptors—the "molecules of emotion"—that control the autonomic nervous system. This means that our heartbeat and blood flow are regulated by our emotions.

Consequently, Candace explained, yoga, meditation, and breath-work practices could be used to bring about concrete changes in the body. For instance, through yoga one can manipulate the emotions, as each posture can trigger feelings that then trigger chemicals that incite immune cells to migrate out of bone marrow to create new tissue. And by using visualization alone, one can increase blood flow to certain parts of the body. Since nutrients are infused and waste products removed with the movement of blood, these surges have curative effects.

Candace also postulated that prayer and meditation strengthen the frontal cortex, the brain's center of "executive functioning," and create feelings of bliss by releasing endorphins and serotonin, the "happiness" neurotransmitter, in the body. This was later found in clinical studies to be true. With examples like these, Candace endorsed thousands of years of Eastern wisdom, legitimizing alternative practitioners and pro-viding practical tools to help people consciously affect which parts of their bodies are active at any given time, teaching them to heal their bodies through their minds and vice versa.

Her message was subversive bordering on heretical, as it defied hegemonies in both religion and medicine. Just as prioritizing a personal relationship with God disintermediates the priest, so encouraging individuals to take charge of their own health sidelines the demigods known as doctors. Her audience was hungry for autonomy, and after decades spent bowing to false idols, Candace felt that she too was channeling the spirit of truth.

CHAPTER TWELVE

THE C-WORD

ODERN SCIENCE DICTATES A DISTINCT SEPARATION OF CHURCH AND LAB, so Candace was reviled where her pious forebears were revered. Once she'd published her exposé of the "sausage-making" aspects of science and veered openly into spiritual territory, she was further shunned by former coworkers.

As Candace transformed publicly from diehard scientist into mind-body guru, many sensed her ambivalence. At mind-body conferences, she was playing to a crowd that adored her, but like Groucho Marx, she didn't want to belong to the club that welcomed her as a member. "I always felt that wasn't really the crowd she wanted love and respect from," says Steve Paul, her NIH administrator. "She'd become fringe, but she never stopped wanting approval and validation from her hardcore scientific peers."

While Candace never found the respect she desired and was now unemployable in science, the mind-body circuit paid her handsomely. Skeptics say that she dove headfirst into this arena because she and Michael were desperate for money after their companies collapsed. She'd landed a $150,000 (nearly $280,000 today) contract with Scribner for her memoir and commanded at least $5,000 per speaking engagement, more than ten times the industry standard for a respected scientist who was not a celebrity. Plus, alternative practitioners didn't care that Candace had failed in the eyes of the scientific community; this only seemed to bolster her status as a renegade savant. She justified their work, so they put her on a pedestal.

Yet Candace's commitment to complementary medicine was certainly genuine. She'd spent years advocating for alternative treatments to be researched and taken seriously at the NIH, and she'd fought valiantly for Peptide T as a nontoxic substitute for chemo-based drugs emerging from the National Cancer Institute to treat AIDS. Wasn't it fair to capitalize now that her ideas had gained traction? The answer would depend on the limits of Candace's ambition.

Candace and Michael's research professorships at Georgetown University School of Medicine had been funded for a decade, and that time was running out. Not to mention that the Peptide T patent, which had been filed by the NIH in 1985, had nearly reached the end of its twenty-year term and, once Eckhart Wintzen withdrew, the couple was again without licensing rights. Their ace card, Michael says, was to come up with new intellectual property and apply for another patent, so he and Candace used their remaining year at Georgetown to solve an issue that had dogged Peptide T from the start. Because their formulation aggregated and lost potency, they created a more stable version of Peptide T called DAPTA in 2005 and filed for a patent that they hoped would become the basis of their next business venture.

The following year, Candace published her second book, *Everything You Need to Know to Feel Go(o)d*, in which she doubled down on her commitment to spirituality, maintaining that "feeling good and feeling God are one and the same." Her speaking fees became the couple's only source of income, so when she received a call from Vivian

Komori, a small business owner and radio show host with a passion for alternative healing, Candace agreed to keynote an event Komori was organizing in California. In preparation, the women spoke often and bonded about being risk-taking entrepreneurs. "We built a fast friendship. I too am a crazy person willing to stick my neck out and do what normal people would never do," Komori says. "Candace and I are both people who jump off a cliff and figure out how to open the parachute on the way down."

Komori also interviewed Candace for her radio show, and she loved that Candace spoke from the heart. "She talked about the power of heart energy, even more than brain energy. She operated from the heart and that's what made her powerful," she continues. "Candace was a very real person. She had to be careful about some of the things she was into—the more 'woo-woo' things—because other scientists would make fun of her, but she really wanted to make a difference."

After the tribute, Candace stayed at Komori's modest adobe ranch house north of Los Angeles in Palmdale, a rural desert landscape of scrub brush, horse farms, Mobil stations, and Denny's, where every other lot is empty. She met Komori's husband, Dennis, whose daily commute to the city often amounted to two hours each way, and their three grown sons, two of whom lived in mobile homes on the property. Over dinner, Candace raved to the Komoris about the wonders of Peptide T, and her stories tugged at their heartstrings; they'd watched a dear friend's son die of AIDS and knew firsthand how vicious the disease could be. And when Candace lamented that she and Michael lacked funds to commercialize her drug, Komori jumped at the chance to contribute.

"My husband and I are working-class people, trying to make ends meet," she says. "We were living hand to mouth, but we wanted to be part of something great." Because the real estate market was high, the

Komoris agreed to take out a second loan on their house in May 2007 and give Candace $250,000 in exchange for 10 percent of the company she planned to form.

As the transaction was under way, Komori was surprised by how anxious Candace seemed, calling every few days to see if the loan had been funded, but she believed Candace's promise to return their money within a year. At the time, Komori hadn't heard of Regulation D, and she didn't know what it meant to be an accredited investor. She's since learned that the Securities and Exchange Commission (SEC) mandates that to invest in a business such as Candace's, she and her husband would need a net worth exceeding $1 million and proof of multiple years of joint annual income of $300,000. Clearly, they didn't meet that threshold. In fact, Komori later realized that while Candace and Michael may have lacked steady salaries after leaving Georgetown, they owned assets worth north of $1 million, including a boat and a second home on Tilghman Island in the Chesapeake Bay, and she wonders why the couple didn't liquidate their own holdings to launch a new company.

Did Candace and Michael understand that accepting Komori's investment may have violated SEC rules? "The majority of little bio-tech companies bomb, but most of the time they don't have good drugs or good management," Michael says now. "You don't get too many shots on goal because these experiments cost millions of dollars." Because Komori's $250,000 wouldn't go very far in the world of drug testing, the couple used her money to pay bills and lease lab space while hunting bigger game, which soon came in the form of a smooth Swiss financier, Michael Laznicka.

Komori remembers the day Candace phoned with exciting news: an intermediary had introduced the couple to a hedge fund manager who wanted not only to invest but also to join their company as chair and CEO. Laznicka had been raised in Switzerland after arriving as a Czech refugee, and he now led Gardner Holding, a global financial fund and consultancy based in Zug. He'd flown out to meet Candace and Michael during July Fourth weekend of 2007 to understand Peptide T's twenty-year trajectory and help them chart a path forward.

Over the days they spent together, Candace and Michael explained that while they hadn't completed safety studies for DAPTA, they believed it was a more effective delivery system for Peptide T and, based on their studies with Peter Heseltine as well as the "Deep Throat" confessions of their trial's investigator, they anticipated that the drug would show antiviral effects in subsequent testing. After a handshake deal, the couple placed their DAPTA patent licenses into a newly formed Swiss company, Rapid Pharmaceuticals AG (the name Rapid stood for Receptor Active Peptides into Drugs as well as for "Ruff and Pert Invent Drugs").

Even if Candace and Michael had tried, they wouldn't have known how to evaluate Laznicka's business acumen. At the NIH, they'd operated in a blissful bubble, as their work was government-funded, and in their previous ventures they'd left the business side to others while they focused on science. Besides, as Michael admits, beggars can't be choosers. The couple wasn't in a position to turn down money, and they understood that Laznicka's funding came with strings attached. In exchange for a 40 percent stake in their joint venture, their benefactor was required to invest $4.1 million ($500,000 initially, followed by monthly infusions of $100,000 for thirty-six months). Candace and Michael would each retain approximately 30 percent for their intellectual property and pull salaries of $12,000 and $10,500 per month for their respective roles as chief scientific officer and research director.

This new accord valued the company at $10.25 million, a fivefold increase over the valuation the couple had agreed upon with Komori just three months prior. Yet somehow Candace and Michael initially neglected to mention Komori's contribution. What's more, when their new CEO learned of it, he attempted to appease Komori by offering 12,500 nonvoting shares and $100,000 of her money back, even though at current valuation her investment was worth more than $1 million.

In January 2008, Komori signed a shareholder agreement attesting that Gardner's $500,000, rather than her previous $250,000, was "first money in." Instead of the 10 percent of Rapid Pharmaceuticals that she'd been guaranteed, Komori now owned a 2.5 percent nonvoting interest. Additionally, because the agreement anticipated that Rapid might need up to $15 million in additional funding to complete foreseen projects, Komori's investment was subject to further dilution. Because she'd already remortgaged her house on Candace's behalf, Komori now lacked the funds to retain a lawyer, and she trusted Candace, Michael, and Laznicka when they portrayed this as a favorable arrangement for all.

By all accounts, Michael Laznicka could be seductive. "He was a bit flash, had a penthouse apartment with all kinds of cars and toys," says Mark Lloyd-Fox, who met Laznicka in June 2008 when the two men were seated together at a friend's fiftieth-birthday party in London. Their hosts that evening had attended a hiking retreat with Laznicka and thought Lloyd-Fox should hear about Rapid because he was HIV positive and thus had a personal interest in a cure.

"[Laznicka] proceeded to show me seminaked pictures of the rentboy who was waiting for him at One Aldwych," Lloyd-Fox says, referring to a five-star hotel in Covent Garden. "Between rentboy stories, he mentioned Candace Pert's name as a potential chief scientific officer and my ears perked up." From his vantage point in London, Lloyd-Fox had heard only positive things about Candace's efforts to supply buyers clubs, and he was curious about how Peptide T compared with antiretrovirals (ARVs). "I had a vested interest in wanting to try it myself."

As Lloyd-Fox recounts, Laznicka believed that the upside at Rapid was larger than the $300,000 per month he'd been earning at Gardner, so he was taking the reins of the company. He offered Lloyd-Fox entry into a "friends and family" investment round in which, he now claimed, the company was valued at a "discounted" $250 million, more than twenty-four times the valuation he'd just agreed upon with Candace and Michael. Soon after, when Laznicka presented him with a financial model professing that Rapid's "true" value would soon exceed $850 million, Lloyd-Fox agreed to become one of eight early investors in the firm. He was in New York on September 15, 2008, when he transferred $500,000 to Rapid's account in Switzerland; it was the same day Lehman Brothers collapsed. "My gut was turning," Lloyd-Fox says, in hindsight. "Maybe that was a sign."

In addition to investing, Lloyd-Fox became vice president of global partnerships and coalitions, which is to say he agreed to leverage his considerable Rolodex to raise money for the fledgling firm. "I have a reasonably good address book," he says. "When I say that, I'm underplaying it. It's a very good one." Lloyd-Fox's birth mother is Ann Lloyd Keen, a British Labour Party politician who served as a member of Parliament from 1997 until 2010 and was married to Alan Keen, a fellow Labour MP who served from 1992 until his death in 2011. Her sister Sylvia Heal was also a Labour MP, as well as a deputy Speaker of the House of Commons, and the family is close with former prime minister Gordon Brown. In addition to royals and moguls, Lloyd-Fox counts among his friends the late actresses Debbie Reynolds and Olivia de Havilland, the bestselling author Ken Follett, and Sir Nicholas Hytner, the former artistic direction of London's National Theatre. He travels in circles of influence.

That wasn't always the case. Like Candace, Lloyd-Fox's mother got pregnant at age nineteen, but she had given up her son for adoption.

He was twenty-eight, working as a director at the Commonwealth Institute in London, when he first reunited with his birth mother, and three years later they collaborated on a public campaign to lower the age of sexual consent for homosexuals in the United Kingdom from twenty-one to eighteen, in line with the age for heterosexuals.

Lloyd-Fox says that he didn't drink until his late twenties and even then he drank only socially, but in January 2000 a three-year relationship ended and he went on a bender of booze and drugs. "There are several weeks I have little account for, and I can only imagine I did not take necessary precautions," he says. "I was cavalier with my normal protections." In November of the previous year, he'd tested negative for HIV as part of a mortgage application for a Covent Garden penthouse—"insurance companies could ask for that information back then"—but when he tested again in July 2000 as part of his annual physical, he received distressing news. "I'd just been part of this very public campaign with my mother, and I realized that if I told a single soul the world would know," Lloyd-Fox says. "I couldn't even tell my best friends. For three and a half years, I kept this dirty little secret to myself."

For a time, Lloyd-Fox suffered from shame, but with treatment he was able to live a relatively normal life, whereas he knew that AIDS remained a death sentence for many around the world. Thus, when he heard about Candace's efforts to bring Peptide T to the masses, he felt aligned in a desire to do well by doing good. "Candace was determined to get this drug out there to as many people as quickly as possible," he says. "This was her life, what she really loved. She wanted to give it away."

After researching the market opportunity for AIDS treatments and understanding their costs, Lloyd-Fox had come to believe that they could make significant margins on Peptide T in the first world while simultaneously offering the drug at low cost in the developing world. He explains that roughly four million people above the equator are infected with HIV, many of whom live in Europe and receive socialized healthcare. However, treatment is denied to many of the twenty-five million AIDS victims in sub-Saharan Africa because these countries' governments have a history of violating pharmaceutical companies' patents on other drugs, choosing to import cheap substitutes from Asia or Pakistan instead. "It's not that they're bloody-minded," Lloyd-Fox says. "They just don't have the money. They can't afford Big Pharma prices." As retribution, pharmaceutical companies withhold access to certain ARVs.

Conversely, Lloyd-Fox envisioned a solution that served both developed and developing world markets. He knew that Rapid could manufacture Peptide T/DAPTA in California for $67 per patient per month, and he estimated that they could sell it for between $250 and $300. "That's 10 percent of the cost of the cheapest ARV, which was at that time $25,000 per year," he says. "Some ARVs cost up to $100,000 per year." Their next step was to determine how much it would cost to make Peptide T in India and research economies of scale. "It came back less than $2 per patient per month for twenty-five million people. With those numbers, we could make it affordable in the West and accessible in the developing world. We could even make a profit just by increasing our numbers, not by increasing the price."

As Lloyd-Fox assessed the global AIDS crisis on a macro level, he also sought to grasp in a micro way what was happening inside his body. He began reviewing his blood work with Candace and learning to read his own charts. "I was hungry to be educated, to increase my knowledge so I could lead my own treatment. Candace taught me," he says. "The breadth and depth of her knowledge was incredible. She could play 3-D chess in her head while stuffing herself with food and having a conversation. I've seen her in rooms full of scientists where they're all writing on the whiteboard and she's stuffing doughnuts in her face, seeming not to pay attention—until she gets up, wipes what they've written off the board, and solves everything."

Candace was riding high on her August 2008 appearance on *Larry King Live* in a segment called "Change Your Mind, Change Your Life." She'd also recently designed a more sensitive PCR test to measure viral reservoirs of HIV in the lymphatic system, the gut, and the brain, where the virus also resides, but which existing tests ignored. While medications such as ARVs restrain the virus, stopping it from replicating and killing host cells, its presence in the viral reservoir never fully vanishes; generally, the virus will surface again on tests, in waves lasting months to years, because it's been hiding there. To treat the viral reservoir and determine Peptide T's effectiveness, Candace first needed a way to quantify it.

Lloyd-Fox began taking Peptide T as a complementary drug alongside his ARVs, and after six months of administering Peptide T nasal spray, his "woefully low" CD4 count, which had hovered around 250 copies per cubic millimeter of blood, increased to 700, and then to 900. According to Candace's new test, after twelve months on Peptide T, Lloyd-Fox was virally undetectable in each reservoir. "We did RNA and DNA tests, and they couldn't find traces of the virus anywhere," he recounts. "We didn't want to use the C-word—*cure*—but it was undetectable."

Against the advice of his clinicians in London, Lloyd-Fox decided to take an "ARV holiday" to try Peptide T as a single-drug protocol, offering himself as a guinea pig to Candace. "Candace said, 'What if it spreads?' But what can spread if RNA and DNA do not show the virus in my body?" he says. "I thought I'd mitigated the risk." In 2009, instead of weaning off ARVs, Lloyd-Fox went cold turkey. Though prevailing science predicted he'd soon be dead, for about four years Lloyd-Fox took monthly trips to Maryland to be monitored and treated only with Peptide T. "There's more of my blood in test tubes in Rockville than there is in my body," he says.

While his first test using solely Peptide T measured no change in Lloyd-Fox's viral load, his second test showed that it had spiked, indicating that the virus was replicating quickly. "Candace was shitting kittens. Mike Ruff and Laznicka were panicking," Lloyd-Fox recalls. "But then they discerned it was dead virus they were finding. When we found that there were no traces in my body other than latent virus, when the genotype was no longer present in my DNA or RNA, and when no blood-brain barrier traces were there either, we still couldn't say it was a cure. Because if you took the test, antibodies would still be present to say I'd had it. But this was showing that all my infected cells would eventually die off according to their natural life span, and then the new cells pumped into my bloodstream from the marrow would be protected. So eventually I wouldn't have HIV anymore. What else would you call it if not a cure?"

Still, one man's miraculous results are not enough to shift the course of medicine. "I don't care about one patient. One has no statistical value. In a Phase III trial, you look at fifteen hundred to two thousand patients and report to the FDA about it. That's how you find out if it's effective," says Jeff Galpin, the Los Angeles–based infectious disease specialist who had investigated Peptide T as a potential cure for PML.

This is precisely what Candace and Michael were trying to do, as they lobbied first for a Phase II clinical trial at the renowned Whitman-Walker Clinic in Washington, D.C., which specialized in HIV. When the clinical director offered them a slot three years hence, Lloyd-Fox thought his results might sway the director into giving them an earlier slot; he turned around his car, drove back to the clinic, and showed the director his tests. It worked. "We were in in two months' time," Lloyd-Fox says. "We jumped the queue massively because they wanted association based on this."

Rapid's management saw dollar signs then and aimed to position the firm for acquisition. They knew that large pharmaceutical companies no longer concern themselves with early-stage research and development, but rather take bets on small biotech companies, scooping them up for, say, $100 million after seeing promising results from a Phase II trial. Big Pharma will then, in turn, absorb the cost of the Phase III trial required to bring products to market. Provided the Whitman-Walker trial produced desired results, Lloyd-Fox and the team envisaged this fate for Rapid. However, he cautioned that Peptide T would be an attractive target *only* if Big Pharma saw it as complementary to ARVs. If pharmaceutical companies got wind that Peptide T functioned as a stand-alone treatment and therefore threatened their existing business in ARVs, these Goliaths would work to squash their David.

"I said, 'Candace, don't think of the Nobel Prize!'" Lloyd-Fox recounts. "We'd be at risk if these firms saw my data. If they found out we were competitive instead of complementary, they could question our results and tie us up in litigation for ten years. We had to keep it under lock and key, at least until we were farther along."

Lloyd-Fox convinced the Whitman-Walker Clinic to agree to position Peptide T as a complementary drug to ARVs, and as the trial got under way he and Laznicka focused on growing Rapid's business, which included considering other uses for Peptide T. The drug had alleviated psoriasis in patients at the Karolinska Institute in Sweden more than twenty years prior, so Candace and Michael wanted to conduct further studies. And because Peptide T appeared to reduce inflammation, as witnessed by Jeff Galpin against his patient's PML, Rapid's management planned to evaluate its effect on arthritis and Alzheimer's disease as well.

As Laznicka and Lloyd-Fox shuttled between London, Zug, New York, and Washington, D.C., they agreed to divide the compounds Candace and Michael had created over time into primary and secondary assets. Rapid's streamlined "mother ship" would hold primary assets (e.g., HIV treatments) that they would continue to nurture in-house, while secondary assets (e.g., treatments for psoriasis, arthritis, and Alzheimer's disease) would be owned by satellite companies that could be sold to pharmaceutical companies that had adequate resources to develop them.

Like Candace and Michael before him, Lloyd-Fox began to seek allies in the government and within powerful AIDS advocacy groups to help Rapid's cause when the time came to unveil the marvels of Peptide T. "Every senator or politician must publish who funds them, from private individuals to Big Pharma or the auto industry. There are five pharma lobbyists for each single member of the House! So I sought to make friends on the Hill with senators like Tammy Baldwin," he says, speaking of the first openly gay woman elected to the House of Representatives and the Senate. "It was clear we'd need the government on our side if the pharmaceutical industry perceived us as a threat and got litigious."

Lloyd-Fox says that he also worked with Regan Hofmann, who was then a senior policy officer at UNAIDS and was, at the time, the editor in chief of POZ, a magazine serving the HIV community. "Regan was in the loop on this and wanted to put it on the front page of everything," he says. "But I said we dare not say anything until our Phase III trial is complete and we're out to market." Additionally, Lloyd-Fox reached out to Kathleen Sebelius, the U.S. secretary of health and human services under President Obama, who had overseen the roll-out of the Affordable Care Act and had previously served as the governor of Kansas, and he began brokering meetings for Candace and Laznicka with the Gates and Clinton Foundations, the Global Business Coalition on HIV/AIDS, and the Global Fund to Fight AIDS, Tuberculosis, and Malaria. "This was big Washington global money," he says. "They wanted to be associated with the release of these data from the trial."

Candace so impressed these organizations' leaders that they began asking her to present to major donors and inviting her and Laznicka to their annual galas. After one such event, a chief executive proceeded to gather five of his top patrons—including two billionaires and the CEO of a telecom conglomerate—at a subsequent meeting in New York. "He took us to his superyacht and said that it's incumbent upon business to find solutions to health crises, positioning [support of Peptide T] as philanthropy with a twist," Lloyd-Fox recounts. "I thought I had to rally the troops. Suddenly I looked up and—suck my buttons—we were surrounded by pretty big names." With support from business and government bigwigs, Candace and Peptide T would triumph at last.

While Candace was "lapping it up," relishing the spotlight at fundraisers on yachts, Lloyd-Fox sensed Laznicka growing wary as he facilitated the company's advance. "His fragile ego couldn't handle it. He hated that I was on the trial as a single drug and was advocating against it," Lloyd-Fox says. "As it became successful, it almost made him worse. I was my own worst enemy in being so gung-ho about it. Each time I came up with a creative scheme, Laznicka got more nervous, like a rabbit in the headlights." Before long, Lloyd-Fox understood why, as some of his "big name" corporate titans performed their own due diligence. Laznicka's background was opaque, they said, making it clear to Lloyd-Fox that they wanted nothing to do with him.

Lloyd-Fox ultimately invested more than $1 million in Rapid, liquidating assets that included his home to move the company forward. As a Rapid employee, he had agreed to accrue his salary and pay his own expenses, accepting reimbursement only when the firm started making money. He believed that Laznicka was doing the same; he'd thought that, as gay men, they were in this together. In February 2010, in good faith, he'd even lent Laznicka $100,000 after several new investors backed out. "He asked me for it, and I gave it to him without a contract," Lloyd-Fox says. "Of course, I didn't get that back, and in October of that year he fired me."

Lloyd-Fox would later learn that instead of providing $4.1 million of his own money, as Laznicka had originally promised Candace and Michael, he'd proceeded to raise $8.85 million from outside sources without diluting his 40 percent stake. According to Gaytri Kachroo, the lawyer tasked with an inquiry, as quickly as Lloyd-Fox could convince his wealthy cohort to invest, Laznicka began siphoning funds. He'd devised a complex, multinational corporate structure that made it impossible for investors to track spending, and he was paying employees in Switzerland and the Netherlands who seemed to play no role in Rapid.

While Rapid's Swiss parent company had transferred the minimum amount required to support the Maryland lab, $7 million had gone missing from the firm on the CEO's watch. As a result, Laznicka was investigated for running a Ponzi scheme to fund his lavish lifestyle; according to Michael, Lloyd-Fox, and Komori, this included a Bentley, male prostitutes, and a $12,000-per-month apartment in London for his Russian boyfriend, as well as first-class flights and presidential suites in hotels around the world.

Laznicka had even launched another Peptide T black market across Europe, peddling an exclusive subscription service with a minimum cost of $50,000. "I had written records of the people Laznicka was distributing to," Kachroo says. "I said, 'Stop right this minute!' I got waivers from everyone who'd taken the drug, waivers saying they wouldn't sue the company if something happened to them as a result, like some side effect."

For months, Lloyd-Fox had been unable to understand why Laznicka wasn't trying to sell or spin off their satellite businesses, as they'd arranged. "I said to him, 'Why are we sitting on cures for psoriasis, neuropathic pain, Alzheimer's?'" Lloyd-Fox says. "As a cure for psoriasis alone, what we had was a way to cure the inflammation that results in flaking skin without any side effect or toxicity. That's a bigger market than HIV!" Indeed, Lloyd-Fox recalls that Laznicka had even tried to stop his single-drug protocol and had argued that Rapid should enroll hundreds of patients in its Whitman-Walker Phase II trial, though the FDA required only a fraction of that number.

Presumably, Lloyd-Fox's test results were garnering the kind of attention Laznicka was keen to avoid, as the due diligence necessary for any potential sale would have exposed the CEO's misdeeds. If Laznicka could keep courting new investors and convince existing investors that they were on the verge of success, then he could conceal both the mislaid funds and his covert drug distribution.

Kachroo's 2012 internal investigation alleged that Laznicka was falsifying data, publishing business plans and promotional documents that obscured the truth. According to the minutes from a Rapid board meeting three years later, while the CEO had been courting investors with a bogus, inflated valuation, he'd known that the firm was more than CHF 2 million (2 million Swiss francs) in debt and at risk of liquidation. Lloyd-Fox and Komori say that Laznicka also bought time by claiming Rapid had conducted clinical trials in Africa but that they'd failed because participants were selling the drugs they were supposed to ingest. "There was always a reason why it was dragging out. He spent a lot of time talking about how crooked it was in Africa," Vivian Komori says. "Then I find out that none of it was true at all. They weren't even doing tests! It was all bullshit, and we bought it hook, line, and sinker."

Upon discovering Laznicka's alleged misappropriation of funds, about a dozen investors flew to Zurich in June for a confrontation, while others joined by phone. As this was going down, Lloyd-Fox was in Wales at the bedside of his adoptive mother, who was dying after a long battle with Alzheimer's. "She's unconscious. I'm holding someone's hand who is squeezing it occasionally, but not really there," he says of his agonizing decision to leave his mother to do battle with Laznicka. "I knew that if she had known I had this pressing matter, she would say, 'Go on, boy.'" When Lloyd-Fox arrived home in London that evening, he learned from his birth mother that his adoptive mother had died. The next morning, he found himself in Zurich, making arrangements with funeral directors hundreds of miles away while scripting his attack on Laznicka.

When Laznicka arrived, he was shocked to find a conference room full of livid investors. "As far as I'm concerned, we're a small, private company. There's a family dispute about to be uncovered and, for now, we're safely inside the home with all the curtains drawn. But outside that door, the FBI is waiting," Lloyd-Fox announced to Laznicka, relishing the metaphor. "On this desk, I have an orange jumpsuit and some KY Jelly—"

"Don't give him the jelly!" shouted another investor, the wife of a dentist from D.C. "I want him to feel it!"

"You have two choices," Lloyd-Fox continued. "Either you wear orange for a long time, or you agree to work with us in a forensic analysis of the company, disclosing everything you have done." In an effort to salvage the company, investors were offering Laznicka the opportunity to come clean. All were stunned when the CEO not only didn't respond to the charges against him but also had the nerve to counter; if investors wanted his help unraveling what he'd done, then they'd have to pay him. Ultimately, Rapid's management chose to settle out of court, so no wrongdoing was ever established, and after a final audit Laznicka retained a minority share of 13 percent. "I wanted him to have a stake in the future success that he couldn't afford to lose or give up on," Lloyd-Fox says. "I didn't want him to sabotage us from the outside."

All the while, Candace and Michael claimed deniability, avowing that, as mere scientists, they lacked oversight and access to Rapid's bank accounts. Investors didn't know then that Laznicka had leverage, for the couple had their own secrets—secrets that tied back to the NIH and which Laznicka had unearthed and was using against them. "Candace and Mike actively participated in bringing him down," Lloyd-Fox says, "yet never exposed their own [complicity]." That would come later.

CHAPTER THIRTEEN

THE TRAVESTY TOUR

INVESTORS HAD BEEN QUESTIONING RAPID'S FUTURE EVEN BEFORE ALLEGATIONS against Laznicka came to light, while the CEO scrambled for ways to save himself and the firm. When Laznicka proposed that Rapid incorporate in the Czech Republic, Candace and Michael had refused because, unbeknownst to shareholders, they were already at war with their CEO.

The couple had agreed to a deal in which Laznicka would receive an additional 1.6 percent ownership of Rapid in exchange for $150,000, which Candace and Michael needed to pay bills. But Candace signed the contract without reading it carefully and only later realized that the decimal point had been omitted. She'd unwittingly handed over 16 percent of her company, clouding its valuation and making Laznicka the majority shareholder. This empowered Laznicka to fire the couple when they opposed him.

"We were like, 'You fucking fired us? Fuck you!'" Michael says. "This was our livelihood, and he was still pulling a salary and driving his Bentley. If he moved our IP [intellectual property] to Prague, it would be beyond our reach. We started looking for a way to dislodge him, which led to the investigation."

Candace's judgment was dubious at that point. Her mania had been intensifying, and as pressure mounted she was becoming unhinged to the point that Mark Lloyd-Fox suspected she was suicidal. "She needed vindication," he says. "She kept saying, '[Peptide T] will help people!'" In 2009, when Lloyd-Fox and Candace went to see the movie *Avatar* with a Czech investor Laznicka was courting, she alienated him by leaping from her seat and screaming at the screen. On a separate occasion, when Lloyd-Fox presented Candace to the son of a Nobel Prize winner, she grabbed the man's arm and cried, "You're gorgeous and amazing! Can I have your sperm? It's for my daughter, Vanessa. You don't have to marry her. You'd just make such good babies!" After a handful of incidents like these, Lloyd-Fox began babysitting Candace at functions and meetings, running interference so that she wouldn't repel supporters.

Candace had also been using food as a sedative, gorging herself regardless of the circumstances, no matter whom she might offend. "She'd get her hair and nails done and within minutes she'd have food all down her blouse and didn't care," Lloyd-Fox recalls. "She would eat all the biscuits and sandwiches in front of her while she was speaking, spitting food all over." To compensate, he began arriving at Candace's hotel room two hours prior to meetings with bags full of food. "I knew she'd be so full that by the time we got to the meeting, she'd actually focus. And then she'd be brilliant."

Even Candace's brilliance wasn't enough to mask her escalating mental illness. While traveling to visit family, she asked a stranger to watch her luggage in New York's Penn Station and then wandered off. When she returned, police had swarmed to check for a possible bomb, and she later had to appear in court for causing a public disturbance.

Candace had even begun to disgrace herself at the paid speaking engagements that had been filling her coffers for years. "The last time she spoke, it was 'the travesty tour,'" says Jane Barrash, the executive director of the Continuum Center, an educational organization in Minneapolis that is dedicated to exploring human consciousness. Barrash had first met Candace in 1988 when Candace spoke at Continuum on the topic "Does Consciousness Survive Death?" and the women bonded over their Jewish heritage. "She was the classic neurotic Jew," Barrash continues. "There were times when she broke down crying about her family, what she grew up with, but mostly she kept it together."

However, the third time Continuum hired Candace to present, she was incoherent and out of control. She'd slipped in the tub prior to coming, so she took the stage in a wheelchair with Michael by her side. "The audience was filled with high-profile people, proper suburban people," Barrash recounts. "She's holding the microphone and makes a joke about holding his penis." Then, at the reception afterward, Barrash whispered to Candace that she had a joint for Michael; because they were all "active pot smokers," this normally wouldn't have been an issue, but Candace drew attention once again by yelling, "He's not supposed to get high anymore!'"

Continuum's board members and donors were appalled, yet Candace seemed unaware of how discordant she appeared and how she'd failed to meet expectations. "Candace was always volatile," Barrash says. "She lived in a dichotomy or at cross-purposes, like a psychologist who goes into a profession because she needs healing. Her most important work was about the role of emotions in our spiritual and physical health, but she was so far from practicing her own message. She was an emotional wreck."

Deborah Stokes, Evan's former nanny who credits Candace with inspiring her career in science, suspects that her mentor suffered from borderline personality disorder. "It's easily triggered into rage and distorted, almost delusional thinking, distorted reactions to things. They launch into extreme emotional reactivity. They are often misdiagnosed as bipolar because of the mania, inability to sleep, heightened sexuality," she explains. "She would often ask me, 'Do you think I was sexually abused? Do I have signs of being sexually abused?'"

After losing touch for years, Stokes had rekindled their relationship when she'd surprised Candace at a conference she was keynoting. Coincidentally, Mildred had died the day before, and when Candace saw her old friend, she broke down crying and thanked her profusely for caring for Evan. The women picked up right where they'd left off, and before long they were inseparable. By then Stokes was getting her PhD in psychology, and she did an internship with Candace at Georgetown University in the department of biophysics. Candace joined Stokes's doctoral committee, and when Stokes went on to study neurofeedback for seventeen years at the Better Brain Center, one of the largest clinics in the United States, Candace would stop by Stokes's office to compare notes. "Forty years later, once I'd made something of my life, she flew across the country for me, to speak to my biology class," Stokes says. "There was not a dry eye in the house when I introduced her, talked about how I was raised, and what she did for me, what she meant to me."

However, by the early 2000s, Stokes was deeply concerned about her mentor. Around the same time Candace spoke at the Continuum Center in Minneapolis, she invited Stokes and her husband, Jim, to stay with her and Michael in California, where Candace was keynoting another conference. "When I tucked her into bed, she was totally hallucinating. She was floridly psychotic, talking to a presence in the room," Stokes recalls. "She'd written one or two papers on bipolar disorder or schizophrenia being an interdimensional phenomenon, saying you can commune with entities on the other side of the veil. That's what she was doing."

Claiming to be in pain, Candace first postponed her talk and requested that Michael again accompany her to the dais. Then, instead of delivering a speech, as planned, Candace instructed Michael to read from her book. "She was so out of it, not tuned into this world," Stokes continues. "People thought she was on drugs." After Candace's onstage escapades, Michael and Laznicka downgraded her role within Rapid and proceeded to block her public speaking engagements. This kept Candace from embarrassing herself and their firm, but it also made her anxious, as she feared being pushed aside.

Furthermore, Candace had become hostile toward Michael's female friends and associates, even those who'd shown no romantic interest. "She had this crazed idea that somehow Mike was interested in me," says her colleague Lydia Temoshok. Tension had begun as early as 1998, when Temoshok worked at the Institute of Human Virology, where Candace and Michael wanted to attend a meeting. Because the $500 ticket price was out of their range, Temoshok offered to make them name tags; in other words, she would sneak them in.

Instead of repaying the favor, however, Candace humiliated her friend. As Temoshok stood beside her poster giving a presentation, Candace made a show of greeting another faculty member. "She said, 'Neil, don't you like my name tag? Do you notice anything funny about it? It's a special name tag!' Then she said, 'Neil, have you met Lydia? She has a perfectly nice husband, but she's always after other people's husbands!'" Temoshok recalls. "This was my first conference there, I'm a new faculty member, and she's shouting about me seducing people's husbands. Also, that men like blondes like me and she doesn't know why. I was mortified."

Late the next night, Candace showed up unannounced on Temoshok's doorstep, brandishing the scissors Temoshok had accidentally left in her car while fashioning the ersatz name tags. When Temoshok peered through her peephole, she became afraid and refused to open her door. "I said, 'Candace, put the scissors down. It's very late at night,'" she recalls. "Her behavior had been crazy." Shortly after, Temoshok received emails from Michael's account saying, "You cold bitch! You cock teaser, stop coming on to me!" "I was like, 'Jesus, why is she doing this?' I knew it was her instead of Mike. I called him and said, 'What the hell is going on? You need to stop her from doing this!'" Temoshok continues. "He told me they shared the same email and said, 'How do you think I feel? I have to work with her.'"

Temoshok distanced herself from Candace then, but by 2002 she was divorced and happily dating another man, so she accepted an invitation to join Candace and Michael for dinner at their house on Tilghman Island. "Candace seemed very reasonable, and I thought, 'Oh, she's normal again,'" Temoshok says. "I'm with Peter and she's with Michael, so she doesn't perceive a problem." However, the women's relationship crumbled again in 2006 when, on the eve of publishing her second book, Candace revealed that she'd falsified a quote from Temoshok.

Candace had written that Temoshok encouraged shouting to release anger, but Temoshok insists she counsels patients toward more appropriate social scripts. When Temoshok offered to substitute words reflecting her true sentiment, Candace refused. "She said, 'You either go with what I have or I'll cut you out,'" Temoshok says. "She was willing to lie—to twist my words and ideas—to make her point!"

Though Temoshok denounces Candace's erratic, unethical conduct, she is quick to note that her distrust of Michael was well founded, as close friends and family believed he'd been cheating for years.

Candace herself presumed as much. In a "highly confidential" stream-of-consciousness "biosketch" detailing her history of trauma that Candace wrote in May 2005 in preparation for *Everything You Need to Know to Feel Go(o)d*, she recounts that Michael "had a brief affair with a prof in our dept! to show he could have an affair anywhere and announced he was going to visit the old gf." At least a year before the Laznicka debacle, Michael had also reconnected with a woman he'd dated in 1980, when he'd been a fellow at the Swiss National Academy of Sciences at the University of Zurich, and Candace suspected that his frequent trips to Switzerland with Laznicka were not work-related.

"I still have her emails talking about Mike's affair," Deborah Stokes says. "She'd come over and cry for more than a year." One morning at 5 a.m., Candace also called Vivian Komori, frantic over letters she'd found in Michael's sock drawer that proved he was cheating. "She was hurting and in shock," says Komori, who realized only later that Candace was complicit in sidelining her investment. "She loved Michael. She was really devastated. My heart breaks because she was so crushed."

Even more troubling, Michael had a habit of touching people without their consent, often in front of his wife. "He'd always say, 'Give me a big hug' and then make sexual comments and put his hands on my hips, grope my ass, or say something about my tits," says Nancy King-caid, Evan's partner. And cousin Nancy Morris reports that Michael asked her tween daughter and niece, "How's your period? Do you have your period yet? Do you feel your boobs developing?" "Michael touched the kids inappropriately. He squeezed their tush," she says. "It only happened once because we never left them alone with him again."

Those closest to Candace also speculated that Michael had been entangled with her sister Wynne. While supervising Peptide T's underground supply, Wynne had been a fixture in the couple's home for a decade, against the advice of other family members. "I did not like Wynne going there. I never felt it was right," Deane says. "Candy was a very powerful person and Wynne was weak. She gave up her painting restoration career because of her mental health issues and then got involved in Candace's work. Wynne lost her identity and was there only to serve Candy and Michael."

As Wynne grew overweight and obsequious, tension between the sisters was palpable. "Wynne didn't have a family, or a boyfriend or husband, or huge success," says Candace's childhood friend Nancy Marriott. "She just kind of shrank away in the shadow, like 'I'm less than, a failure.' Candace was taking full advantage, like 'I am the queen, and you are the servant.'" Marriott recalls that while attending a party with the sisters at a posh politico's home in Washington, D.C., Candace started berating Wynne because she'd disagreed with her point of view. "I intervened and said, 'Candace, stop! You can't talk to your sister like that!' It was so nasty. It was public; there were people around us overhearing. Wynne shrank and shrank and shrank, and I felt sorry for her."

Others attributed the sisters' strain to Michael and Wynne's flirtatious relationship. "Wynne was meek and very fragile, on the verge of being in a mental ward, and Michael was dominant over her," Evan says. "He was flirty with her. He's a very touchy-feely, trolly guy. He'd grab her ass and touch her. There could have been sexual engagement." Even Candace suspected her husband was cheating with Wynne. In the same "biosketch" in which she'd recorded Michael's affairs with his Swiss girlfriend and a professor in their department, she wrote that "he may have had some form of sex with my sis (which he always denied)—he bragged of it in email to old gf which I intercepted."

After two prior suicide attempts, Wynne was found dead in the bathtub of her apartment in 1998. At her funeral, some found it curious when Michael penned a "Love Remembrance" that was distributed as part of the memorial pamphlet. "Those who we love remain with us, for Love itself lives on, and cherished memories do not fade because of death," he wrote. "Those who we love will never be more than a thought apart from us, for as long as we remember you Wynne, you will live on in our hearts and in our lives."

Based on many conversations with Michael, Lydia Temoshok is convinced he had an affair with Wynne, as she recalls him divulging their "inappropriately intimate" bond. "He more or less confessed that he'd had an affair," Temoshok says. "After Wynne committed suicide, he admitted to me that he'd had a relationship and said maybe her suicide was related to guilt. He talked about the closeness they had, and I think Candace suspected it. Mike probably was cheating on her with various people, and she suspected that. I think a lot of Candace's paranoia was rooted in reality."

As Temoshok indicates, mental health is a spectrum, and Candace was genetically predisposed to a certain type of illness. Yet, as Candace demonstrated in her work, stress plays a meaningful role in physical and emotional well-being, and one cannot help but wonder whether the duplicity and gaslighting she endured in both her personal and professional lives pushed her over the edge. Was Candace born this way, or had she been driven insane?

Before long, Candace was institutionalized again. Michael was en route to Switzerland when Evan received a call from his mother's housekeeper begging him to help. Evan raced to Candace's Potomac home and found her in the backyard, lying in her nightgown under a bush and salivating, foaming at the mouth. "She growled at me like an animal," he says. "I said, 'Mom, it's me, Evan—your son.' And she said, 'You're not my son. You have a mask on.'"

Michael returned from the airport and together they sped to the hospital, but when they stopped at a traffic light Candace jumped out of the car, charged into an intersection, and had to be wrestled back inside the vehicle. "At Georgetown [University Hospital], she was nuts. She started yelling that she wanted a beer, and she never drank beer," Evan remembers. "They put leather straps on her and started injecting her. It's the most horrible thing I can remember. She was screaming. She was tortured mentally by her own demons, and by Michael with this other woman."

When asked about his affairs, Michael does not admit a relationship with Wynne, but concedes that he sought escape from Candace's tyranny. "I said, 'I'm not going to stay married to you anymore. It's too much,'" he says. "'Don't kick the door in. Don't pick up a knife and chase me across the house. Don't threaten to kill yourself.'" Michael says that Candace, in her bipolar delusion, had started throwing phones across the room at board meetings. He also recalls a conference in Australia at which he was speaking when his wife mounted the stage, pushed him out of the way, and grabbed the microphone. "I'm there humiliated, but she's pontificating? I couldn't take it anymore.

"It was a firework that would explode and dissipate," Michael continues. "Working together closely, it never stopped. At 3 a.m., she'd wake me up: 'I have an idea!' She would never relent. It just escalated; if she was a one, I came back with one point five, she'd come back with a two. How far could we crank up the dial? I would never win an argument. Some of those ended up with doors being kicked in. She would do whatever it took to get what she wanted. But we didn't hold grudges or resentments. Every night we'd fall into bed in each other's arms and clear the deck."

By the time they launched Rapid, Candace and Michael fought openly all the time. They made no attempt to hide that they were at each other's throats, even in front of friends and work associates, who attest that while Candace adored Michael, she also brutalized him. "Mike took her abuse," Deborah Stokes says. "To see them interact, I never saw anything but resignation when she would scream and berate him. He would just duck his head down, cower in the corner, and ignore her, which drove her nuts." When the couple visited Stokes's Delaware beach house, Candace sunbathed nude in the yard before initiating a screaming fight with Michael in the street, after which Stokes received calls from neighbors forbidding her from ever hosting the couple again.

"She didn't treat anyone else that way, except maybe her kids and Agu. Mike appeared to really love her, but I think she made him crazy. I'm sure he had such compressed rage," Stokes continues. "I imagine his adrenals are totally shot from the inconsistency, the up and down, the unpredictability of her. She was so fucking intense. I think it wore him out."

Why didn't Michael leave Candace, then? Stokes believes that he was "always looking for a mother," as he'd been born out of wedlock in Ireland and raised in an orphanage until age four, when he was adopted by his American family. "Who knows what happened to him early on? It was always messy with him and Candace—these two brilliant, flawed humans. The amount of stress they withstood for so many years was incredible. They lived in a cyclone, a blender that was constantly on, both of them caught up in a constant folie à deux—enmeshed, entrenched, codependent, screaming, shouting, spring-loaded love-hate. It would have killed anyone."

Jane Barrash also witnessed Candace's haranguing and felt sorry for Michael. He seemed a doormat or punching bag, beleaguered by his wife's cutting remarks. "Candace was brilliant, but she sabotaged everything," she says. "Of course, she attracted all the wrong people, and of course, there's going to be drama. Mike had to deal with the fallout of her drama."

Yet Candace also adored Michael and was desperately afraid to lose him, and her family believes he preyed upon this insecurity. Candace gave her husband credit for her discoveries and seemed preoccupied with his success, often at the expense of her own. For the sake of her marriage, she was willing to sacrifice her money and talents to elevate Michael. "She didn't want him to leave her, so she'd say, 'Michael's so great!'" Evan says. "That's why he still has credibility with people, because of all that pumping up. People treat him like a saint for staying with her and taking care of her. He gets rewarded for being the nursemaid."

According to Candace's children, by playing the victim and assuming the role of their mother's long-suffering caretaker, Michael elicited sympathy from outsiders. They say that though he appeared sheepish, he would morph behind closed doors. Evan and his partner, Nancy Kingcaid, observed that Candace seemed steady and cheerful when Michael was absent, and they became convinced that he was provoking emotional outbursts. "According to my mom, he'd instigate and then act like she just went nuts," Evan says. "He basically let her look like the total crazy one, but he drove her crazy."

Others claim he could be verbally and emotionally abusive. "Michael said the most painful things," says Nancy Morris. "He was always degrading. He would put her down, saying she was overweight and not attractive sexually." One Thanksgiving, Morris recounts overhearing Michael tell his wife, "Look at you, your body. You should be ashamed of yourself. How could I go to bed with you, you're so big?" Similarly, Lydia Temoshok says Michael confided to her that "their sex life was terrible, that he wanted to divorce [Candace], and that she was threatening to take him to court. He said, 'She's always trying to have sex with me, and I can't do it anymore. I don't want to touch her!' He told me that he said to her, 'I don't find you attractive at all and I don't want to have sex with you.' It was so disturbing."

As Rapid foundered, Candace's family knew that her marriage was in trouble, but they didn't realize the extent of the couple's antipathy until Evan and Kingcaid stopped by Candace's home one afternoon to borrow a power washer and overheard Michael raging in the backyard. "He was yelling at my mom, and she was saying, 'Please, Michael. No, no, no!'" Evan says. "He didn't know we were there. We listened to him yelling for ten minutes. . . . I'd never seen him hit her, but he had a rage we'd seen—a whole other side that existed."

CHAPTER FOURTEEN

FIGHTING VIPERS

A S A THIRD COMPANY TEETERED ON THE BRINK OF DISASTER, EVERYTHING ASSO-
ciated with Peptide T felt cursed. "Candy felt rejected by Michael
and also had her drugs rejected," Nancy Morris says. "I remember
her telling me once, 'Don't let these guys push you around in your
career. Look what they've done to me.'" Despairing that her life's work
would be pilfered and destroyed by mercenary men, Candace sought
to align with a powerful woman who might salvage Rapid from immi-
nent demise.

Lawyer Gaytri Kachroo arrived at just the right time, and she
appeared to be the pit bull Candace needed to grapple with Laznicka.
Kachroo had made her name as a partner and international practice
chair at the Boston office of law firm McCarter & English, representing Harry Markopolos, the whistleblower who'd spent a decade badger-
ing federal regulators to investigate Bernie Madoff's fraud. If Kachroo
had taken on Madoff, Candace reasoned, she could no doubt unseat
Rapid's CEO. "Candace was all about women by then," Michael says.
"Candace thought of Gaytri as an ass-kicker like she was. Gaytri was
going to be a hero for us."

With bankruptcy looming yet again, Candace and Michael put full faith in this latest "savior," hiring Kachroo as their personal lawyer in March 2012. At first she seemed to deliver. It was Kachroo who led the investigation that exposed Laznicka's alleged malfeasance, and after orchestrating the strike in Zurich she negotiated a new master agreement to restructure Rapid Pharmaceuticals AG that summer. At that time, Laznicka (through his holding company Gardner) owned 54.15 percent of total equity, having sold 3.35 percent of his stake to forty-one participation certificate holders (PC investors), while Candace and Michael together owned 41.5 percent and Vivian Komori owned 1 percent. In addition to being the firm's CEO, Laznicka was its sole board member.

Kachroo's agreement acknowledged that disputes between the firm's major shareholders were being resolved to reflect the contributions of all parties so that the company could capitalize on investments and pharmaceutical joint venture opportunities. Gardner AG agreed to place 15 percent of its shareholding in Rapid AG (thirty-five thousand shares and forty thousand participation certificates, or 7 percent of all outstanding voting shares and 8 percent of participation shares) into a trust or escrow account to be managed by Kachroo Legal Services (KLS) or the law firm White and Case and supervised by Rapid AG in order to effect an immediate adjustment to Candace and Michael's shares "as a correction of previous transactions and in recognition of the settlement of various conflicts between the parties." In exchange, Candace and Michael would pay Gardner AG $189,000 for services rendered and to settle conflicts.

Both Gardner AG and Candace and Michael consented to an adjustment to PC investors' holdings based on their contributions. By the terms of this new contract, Candace and Michael would now own 55 percent of Rapid AG and Laznicka (via Gardner AG) would be left with 13 percent, while PC investors and Vivian Komori would increase their shares to 30 percent and 2 percent, respectively. When Kachroo also swooped in with a cash commitment from outside investors, to be delivered only after Laznicka stepped down, Candace and Michael credited her with saving Rapid and enabling them to oust their CEO once and for all.

"We had prevailed, gotten Laznicka out, and our girl was going to come in with millions!" Michael says. As far as Candace and Michael were concerned, Kachroo alone would wield the sword of justice against Laznicka.

Of course, justice came at a price. Because Candace and Michael had been unable to pay Kachroo's $650-per-hour legal fee, their lawyer's engagement letter of March 27, 2012, stated that in exchange for a reduced hourly rate plus any expenses and costs incurred, KLS would receive 5 percent of founders stock in Rapid AG (to dilute proportionally with the other founders) for acting on Candace and Michael's behalf, to vest 2 percent the first year, 1.5 percent the second year, and 1.5 percent the third year of service. This equity was awarded on top of a stipend of $100,000 upon the company's anticipated capital raise of $6 million. Beside Candace's signature on this contract, she wrote "Yes!" and drew a heart.

Kachroo's restructuring agreement also instructed that an interim board would be appointed at an extraordinary general meeting of shareholders and would consist of herself (counsel and development); her brother Lee Kachroo, a former banker who'd conducted a forensic review of Rapid's books (finance); and Jiri Chroustovsky, a representative of prominent Czech investors (corporate governance and accounting). These three interim board members would be considered independent contractors, rather than employees of Rapid AG, and were to serve in their capacities for no less than three and no more than six months, or until a permanent board was in place. While no member of the interim board would be eligible to sit on the company's permanent board, they would be permitted to join Rapid AG's management team.

As a result, Candace and Michael agreed that Lee Kachroo would be appointed interim chief financial officer and then a strategic consultant to the company, while Gaytri Kachroo would become general counsel in August 2012, earning CHF 240,000 annually. A month prior, Candace and Michael had relinquished 30 percent of their own stake in Rapid, which amounted to a 17 percent interest in the firm, in exchange for her legal services. Even though Candace and Michael's share was subject to dilution by new investments, they agreed that Kachroo's stake was not.

At the time, Kachroo was still operating as Candace and Michael's personal attorney. On July 27, 2012, to address a potential conflict of interest, she emailed the couple a letter avowing that should she become general counsel of Rapid AG, her interests would remain aligned with Candace and Michael, with whom she would consult on all management and operational matters. She stated that, based on Rapid's current valuation of $35 million, she anticipated selling 10 percent of shares through PNR Holdings (Candace and Michael's investment vehicle, with PNR standing for "PertNRuff") for $3.5 million; of that, $1 million would be set aside for Candace and Michael personally, $1 million would be loaned to Rapid AG, and the final $1.5 million would pay both Laznicka and expenses incurred by Kachroo's and her brother's respective holding entities. This included expenses from Kachroo Legal Services.

The next day, Kachroo sent an additional "Full Disclosure and Potential Conflict Waiver Letter" reiterating that there were no conflicts of interest in her acting as Candace and Michael's personal attorney while also attempting to become general counsel and secure an equity stake in their firm. She did, however, grant that her interests might diverge from theirs at some point in the future. Even though her own master agreement stated that, as a member of the interim board, Kachroo was ineligible to serve on the firm's permanent board, she never relinquished her seat. Instead, she was positioned to replace Laznicka as Rapid's next chair and CEO, in addition to continuing in her role as general counsel.

While Candace and Michael supported Kachroo, they lacked sufficient power to spirit her through the company's front doors. So, according to Padma Oza, Rapid's administrator, who also oversaw Candace's personal accounts, the couple sold $300,000 in stock, plus their home on Tilghman Island, to purchase a greater percentage of Rapid and then leveraged their influence to elevate Kachroo.

Such an appointment required buy-in, however, and not all of Rapid's shareholders saw Kachroo as the perfect fit. Yes, she was a successful executive who had helped them in their time of need, but she lacked proficiency in patent law, had never run a biotech company, and was ignorant about science and venture capital. Surely there were better candidates to steer Rapid into port.

Candace, however, was adamant that Kachroo be installed. She and Michael didn't balk even when one of Rapid's investors, Stephen Kennedy Smith, the son of former ambassador to Ireland Jean Kennedy Smith and the nephew of a former U.S. president, moved to block Kachroo based on their personal entanglement. "Stephen had a relationship with Gaytri," Michael says, elaborating that they were both from Cambridge, Massachusetts, and had been romantically involved long before either one became engaged in Rapid. "When she was trying to come into the company, [Stephen] advised Candace against it."

None of this raised a red flag about Kachroo's fitness to lead the firm? "Candace didn't check too deeply into her background and neither did I," Michael acknowledges. "Gaytri came recommended by a guy who was SVP at Pfizer. We needed the battle to be taken on, and she was ready to take it on."

For her part, Kachroo says that, as a celebrated lawyer with a lucrative practice, she never aspired to be Rapid's CEO, but relented when Candace begged her to take the top job. "I interviewed one CEO after another in the biotech field before I agreed, and that was only after I'd put my own money into the company," she says. "Candace and Mike wanted me on that board. They controlled 55 percent of the company through PNR Holdings, so PNR was running the company. They voted me in."

In a June "Agreement Among Certain Members and Affiliates of PNR Holdings, LLC" drafted by Kachroo, she stated that the anticipated $5 million investment she would procure entitled her to up to 20 percent ownership interest in Rapid AG. She also provided that her legal bills for services to Candace and Michael (PNR Holdings) had been submitted to Rapid AG for payment.

Within the year, Kachroo, via her Anguilla-based holding company Venus Corporation, owned 37.5 percent of Candace and Michael's investment vehicle PNR. By then she had not only raised funds from others but also contributed $400,000 of her own money and accrued another $100,000 in expenses. "Candace and Mike didn't pay me. They didn't give me any of their own equity. The only equity I got came from Laznicka when we restructured," Kachroo explains. "They also didn't pay my costs. I footed the bill for traveling around the world as part of the Laznicka lawsuit."

Candace and Michael had hired outside counsel who approved these deals on the basis that Kachroo did not own shares directly in

Rapid. Rather, she was a minority, nonvoting shareholder in PNR, the holding company owned by the couple. Either way, Candace celebrated Kachroo's ascent to chair and CEO as a girl-powered win. "Gaytri and Candace would joke that they'd run off and be Thelma and Louise," says Nancy Kingcaid. "I looked at Candace one time and said, 'You know they die at the end of that movie, right?'"

In summer 2013, Kachroo's investor, Cynthia Ingraham, the ex-wife of a billionaire hedge fund manager and philanthropist, was ready to infuse Rapid with much-needed cash. Because Ingraham was also her legal client, Kachroo knew that she was passionate about finding a cure for autism, and so she had presented Peptide T to Ingraham as a potential treatment. In August, Kachroo drafted an agreement for Ingraham to invest $1.5 million in Rapid's wholly owned subsidiary focused on autism spectrum disorder (ASD) research and development, with $500,000 to be used in current Rapid programs, including a Phase I trial, and $1 million allocated to the ASD silo. The contract gave Ingraham the option to invest another $1.5 million, for a total of $3 million, which could be directed toward the ASD silo as well. This pact stated that its parties expected to apply a valuation of or around $30 million for the company in determining the shares issued for Ingraham's capital investment.

Ingraham, who had made the entire $3 million placement by the end of 2014, would later accuse Kachroo of violating their contract by using her money for other purposes and never disclosing conflicts of interest. Indeed, while Candace had previously speculated about Peptide T's effect on autism and Kachroo subsequently made legitimate efforts toward clinical trials, no ASD silo existed within Rapid AG at the time of Ingraham's investment and, according to court allegations, the firm never moved to create an ASD silo and spent less than $200,000 on autism trials. "I drove with Gaytri to Cynthia's home in The Boltons and she said, 'I feel conflicted,'" Mark Lloyd-Fox recounts. "I told her, 'You should. It's clearly a conflict of interest.' I told her not to take Cynthia's money, but she did it anyway. Gaytri is incredibly clever, but she too has been tarnished by greed."

Michael later alleged that Kachroo's savvy solution served her own interests at her clients' expense; he accused her of charging Rapid AG for legal work she'd done for the couple personally and attempting to pocket up to $1.5 million of Ingraham's investment. But Kachroo insists their arrangement presented no conflict, as she'd billed only for associates at KLS. "I had four or five attorneys and paralegals working on this 24/7," she says. "I don't have one legal invoice paid by Rapid. At the end, Rapid owed KLS about $2.5 million, and none of that was paid."

Candace and Michael seemed to be magnets for opportunists— or, as Vivian Komori says, "birds of a feather." Even before the Laznicka inquiry, Candace was spiraling and in no condition to make business decisions. She appeared intent on repeating the same mistakes, failing to research the backgrounds of potential partners and employees before hiring them or to set explicit terms at the outset of engagements. By selling her assets to install Kachroo as chair and CEO, she'd made yet another reckless move out of desperation. Anyone seemed preferable to Laznicka and, lacking financial expertise, Candace and Michael had come to believe they needed Kachroo to succeed. And because Kachroo had managed to appease their investors and imbue Rapid with much-needed cash, Candace continued to sing her praises. "Candace loved Gaytri, gave her a round of applause," Deborah Stokes says. "But with Candace, you were either a love or a hate object. There was no in-between with her. She would fawn over people, but she could turn on a dime."

If Candace was suspicious when Kachroo installed her brother as CFO and her son Kirin as comptroller, she kept it quiet within the firm. Yet as Candace's mania heightened so did her paranoia. "She had Michael handle all the money and bills, even in restaurants. She wouldn't sign any checks. She wouldn't put her signature on anything," Evan says. "If something bad was going on, she didn't want to be a part of it. Maybe she knew but didn't want to know. The road to hell was paved with my mom's good intentions."

However, when Padma Oza, who with Michael was responsible for Rapid Lab's payroll and accounting, complained to Candace that Kachroo's son had demanded her password to access funds under Oza's name, Candace could no longer claim ignorance. "I told Candace that if he uses my password and does something wrong, I could be blamed for it," Oza says. "Candace told me, 'You have to protect yourself.' She said whatever they were telling me, I should make a copy. 'Do you have anything in writing?' she said. I contacted the bank and said we need a third person to be signatory."

As for Michael, he seemed out to lunch. Oza says that while Laznicka was CEO, she'd begged Michael to access the parent company's bank accounts in Switzerland. As treasurer of Rapid Labs, a subsidiary of Rapid AG, Michael had only limited access to funds, and Oza wanted to know why Laznicka sometimes sent Rapid Labs less than needed to cover monthly expenses. Yet even after reports that Laznicka had been using the firm's money as his personal slush fund, Michael made no effort toward oversight.

"I told him so many times, 'Mike, at least ask for the password!'" Oza says. "Gaytri's son and brother had it. Candace asked him too." But, according to Oza, Michael refused. "Candace would have been better without Mike than with Mike. He was not doing much, work-wise. Mike was lazy. The amount of power and energy Candace was showing, he was not doing one-tenth of it. I said, 'Candace, your mind is not working. Your mind is upside down.' The amount of stress she was taking, Mike was careless."

Michael admits to being distracted at that time. "In 2013, I was prepared to let my wife shoulder the burden because it was easier for me," he says, recalling that Candace spent hours in tears, screaming on the phone with Kachroo. "She was susceptible to being undermined. As cocky as she was, if you could find the soft spot, you could weaken her. Candace was under a lot of stress and there was a lot at stake."

Somehow, despite these calamities, Rapid's business appeared to be improving. Kachroo had agreed to follow the strategy Lloyd-Fox laid out, and as a result, he says, Rapid soon had preliminary bids of $80 million, $60 million, and $40 million from large pharmaceutical companies for three of its compounds. However, Lloyd-Fox recommended that, before proceeding with a sale, Rapid conduct its own formal due diligence process to ensure it had left no stone unturned. "We'd already had the Laznicka scandal and managed to keep that in-house. Now we needed proper governance," he says. "We needed to know what companies would find when they looked into our operations. Who would buy a house without a surveyor?"

This seemed an obvious and prudent request, so Lloyd-Fox was shocked when Michael initially tried to block an investigation. In turn, Lloyd-Fox reminded him that the minutes from their meeting would be distributed to shareholders. If companies failed to move forward with Rapid and a sale was undermined because the management team had hidden something, then lawsuits would follow. But what could they be hiding?

The night of September 11, 2013, Candace sent Lloyd-Fox a Skype message saying that she needed to discuss an urgent matter; she knew things would be uncovered in an investigation and wanted to explain.

The following day at 12:43 p.m. EST, Candace sent an email to friends and potential investors, with Michael and Kachroo cc'ed. It read:

Dear Friends~

Yup my mind has finally broken free of the prison of helplessness and blame in the face of Evil- thanks to Gaytri!

She has managed to take over Rapid Pharmaceuticals, AG on behalf of Mike and me (PnR Holdings, LLC) and raise several million dollars dedicated to curing autism. The new (Impressive) Board is officially installed by the Shareholders at a meeting in Zurich last week, meeting today for the first time and Gaytri is officially Chairman & CEO.

Michael Laznicka is now a minority shareholder without any power, but I know some of his immoral and viper-ish activities have caused a loss of interest in RAPID while he is involved in any way. So today I share information Gaytri provided me recently.

Laznicka would be willing to part with all his shares for 1M$, well below the current valuation. You should also know that all past debts incurred by RAPID AG while he was CEO are being settled and paid out as funds are available. (I am thinking of Russ Mason's claim for example-he has not been in touch for a long time).

As for me? I am feeling ecstatic but ill these last few days hard to breathe with a pneumonia being treated with antibiotics. Fighting vipers is hard work even from the sidelines! [but] probably just from talking on the phone too much!

Next Thursday/Friday there are meetings scheduled at the lab with professional Pharma experts from the board to chart the new RAP clinical trials being funded, with much related new investment in process. At last professionals are helping us to monetize the medicines to come from inventions Mike and I have made through all these years! If there is any interest in helping in the final slaying of the viper as outlined here, please contact Gaytri or me soonest. Thanks for all your help and encouragement along the way!

My best,
Candace
Candace Pert, PhD
RAPID Pharmaceuticals, AG
Chief Scientific Officer & Director
RAPID Laboratories Inc.
15010 Broschart Rd.
Rockville, Maryland 20854

Less than an hour later, Candace was dead.

CHAPTER FIFTEEN

COMING CLEAN

"**A** PATENT CAN HAVE MISINFORMATION IN IT BUT IT'S STILL VALID. IF HALF IS garbage and half is true, then the claims are still golden," says Evan, who was a primary patent examiner for eighteen years. "My mom was like a patent in that way; she could spout things that are garbage, and things that are genius." Candace's garbage didn't negate her genius, however, and many seemed keen to capitalize.

Four days after Candace died, Kachroo—who had been CEO for all of two weeks—wrote a letter to "All Rapid Shareholders and Friends" that some read as an attempt to fortify power. "Her death, albeit of natural causes (she had been complaining of ill health in the past few days) comes as a great shock to us all and leaves a great void in our hearts," Kachroo writes. "Due to the family's wish that the information remain private including the plans of her cremation, and private ceremony honoring her worldly spirituality, this information was not disseminated earlier."

Kachroo then explains that she and Candace had spoken from approximately 3:30 to 5:30 p.m. on Wednesday, September 11, 2013, during which time Candace "was excited and looking forward" to board meetings the following week. She also assures readers that Candace had "a peaceful mind, and that she was satisfied that RAPID was headed for great success . . . success to which she had dedicated and sacrificed her life." Kachroo then uses the same strange term again, writing that Candace's "life was a sacrifice in the name of healing, and I, along with RAPID's new Board, assure you all, it was not in vain . . . it has become clear that Candace surrendered to the other side only when she was assured in her mind that this Company was finally and optimally positioned for success."

Needless to say, those closest to Candace were unnerved. Candace had anything but a peaceful mind. And who was Kachroo, who had known Candace for less than two years, to pass judgment on her existence, declaring it a sacrifice? Who was she to speak for Candace in life, much less utter her intentions from the grave?

Given the fires Kachroo was fighting at Rapid, she portrayed herself as Candace's anointed one, embarking on a charm offensive and soliciting support. In the wake of Candace's death, Kachroo tried to curry favor with family and friends, particularly those who were useful to Rapid, and some observed that she used Candace's memorial service as an opportunity to network. "My sister dropped dead with no warning and Gaytri spent the whole time on her phone, talking about the business and money, being officious on her iPad," says Candace's sister Deane. "She was so self-promoting and just looking for opportunities. I said, 'Give us twenty-four hours to grieve!'"

Likewise, Andrea Schara, a Bowen family systems therapist who was close with Candace for decades, says that "Gaytri wasn't going to miss an opportunity to make friends with everybody. She could put the full-court press on you. She was a very seductive, good-looking woman who somehow made Candace feel safer, but at the expense of her trust of Mike." Schara had been leery of Kachroo for some time, after hearing from Candace that this new CEO was driving a wedge between her and her husband. The couple's relationship was already strained and distant, and she believes that Kachroo pitted them against each other in a bid for power. "She really got in under Candace's skin and did a number on her, I think."

Schara, who for eighteen years was on faculty at Georgetown Family Center, likens the triad controlling Rapid to Adam, Eve, and the snake in the Garden of Eden. "Mike was not the most thorough, detail-oriented business guy and he'd had an affair. Candace wanted to control Mike more than Mike wanted to be controlled. They had a relationship that's not steady enough to manage the stress," she says. "Gaytri succeeded at getting Candace on her side against Mike. It was always two against one. Gaytri was playing on Candace's vulnerability."

From Kachroo's perspective, however, it was Candace who'd dominated their relationship. After feeling diminished by Michael and Laznicka, Candace wasn't about to let this happen again; instead, she sidelined her husband and cemented herself as Kachroo's sole point of contact. "A real sisterhood grew out of that," Kachroo says. "She said, 'Gaytri, you're the woman I was never able to be. I had three kids and there was no way I could have raised them alone. You didn't depend on a man. You did it on your own.'" Michael was excluded from the women's daily phone calls and didn't accompany his wife on visits to Cambridge. As a result, Kachroo says, she had almost no contact with Michael until after Candace died. "Candace said she wanted to protect me from Mike," Kachroo continues. "She said Mike was into the money."

For the sake of Rapid's future, Michael and Kachroo initially presented a united front, highlighting Candace's brilliance and downplaying her dysfunction. Some say they conspired to design a memorial service that paid tribute to an idealized Candace, with an eye toward protecting their company's interests. Indeed, instead of grieving the loss of his wife, Michael seemed more interested in leveraging Candace's legacy to promote Rapid.

Lydia Temoshok, the psychologist who'd been a friend of the couple's for decades, recounts that when she heard of Candace's death, she visited Michael to lend support, but became uneasy when he rattled off a list of luminaries he wanted to speak at her memorial, including Deepak Chopra, Sol Snyder, and the head of the NIMH. "I said, 'Mike, it's a memorial. You have to bring in the family and other friends who knew her,'" she says. "I wanted to honor her, but he seemed all about the business—using the memorial as a chance to promote it. At the service, it was crass, financially related: *We want her work to go on! Donate here!*'"

In the end, Candace's friends and family appreciated that Chopra and Snyder both headlined the event, as these men formed the bookends of Candace's life, underscoring her fusion of science and spirituality. What shocked them, however, was Kachroo's prominent role. "Gaytri demanded that I let her speak and I did, which I regret," Michael says. "A lot of people said she was working the crowd to collect names, numbers, and contacts to invade my life. . . . There were a lot of directed, pointed questions about why she was trying to insert herself. Some of the women and even Agu remarked on it."

In a sordid leitmotif, Michael and Kachroo each claim that the other made advances shortly after Candace died. "We'd been spending time together, having business meetings and talking about the company. One night we were drinking wine and talking at a bar, and she said, 'You're a cute guy. You should get women,'" Michael recounts. "She made it clear to me that if I was interested in taking her home, she was up for it. It wasn't overtly spoken, but it was a message that was indicated and received. I just felt, 'This is really not right.' She was still my CEO, so no way that was going to happen." Kachroo balks at this accusation and says it was the other way around.

Regardless, following Candace's death, Kachroo drafted employment contracts in May 2014 providing payment to herself of CHF 360,000 per year as CEO and CHF 120,000 per year as chair, plus bonus and stock options, on top of a $25,000-per-month retainer for her law firm. This agreement also included a "golden parachute" of no less than three years of salary and fees should she be terminated.

Additionally, Kachroo, along with her brother and son, consolidated control over the company's finances. By then she'd discovered that Rapid Labs was $150,000 in debt to the federal government because, for at least four years, management had failed to pay payroll taxes, which Padma Oza didn't know was part of her job. Though Oza comes from a family of shrewd businesspeople and studied accounting in college in India, she'd never worked as an accountant in the United States. So when Candace and Michael hired her to be their administrator, she didn't understand the liability associated with her role.

"Mike gave me his password to do whatever with the money. At home, in my father's business, if someone gives you this much power, they trust you so much," Oza says. "But there was money in Switzerland I couldn't see. They told me to sign checks, but I didn't know that being a signatory meant I was responsible to pay for the tax also." After learning that Michael owned a million-dollar house in Potomac and had nearly that amount in his personal bank account, authorities placed three liens on his residence. Two were filed by the state of Maryland in December 2013 and February 2017 for $21,292 and $3,991, respectively, while the IRS is listed as creditor on a third lien for $82,734 in July 2015.

Because Kachroo was unaware that Candace and Michael had given Oza access to their email, the administrator says she intercepted messages in which Kachroo wrote freely about evading the IRS. "The IRS was going to look for Gaytri's money too, and she knew I knew everything. She was scared of me. That's why she wanted me out of the picture," Oza recounts. "They were going to Switzerland at that time— Gaytri, Mike, and her son, trying to hide our accounts in Switzerland. They were talking about filing for bankruptcy and if they did, I would know what they were doing. After Gaytri fired me, I told the federal officer I didn't have access to anything anymore."

In the minutes from a board meeting on March 23, 2015, Kachroo asserts that while Rapid AG, the Swiss parent company, provided the majority of Rapid Labs' funding, "we have gone through a lot of trouble and expense to make sure the entities are distinct from each other." Though Oza paints this attempt to distance Rapid Labs as a strategy to shield the parent company's Swiss accounts from the IRS, Kachroo says she was never responsible for Candace and Michael's gaffes.

"Mike was the treasurer, and he'd been ignoring messages from the IRS. . . . In late 2014, my son saw there were IRS invoices, and then notices. It was a big deal," she explains. "As soon as I took over, we were paying payroll taxes. But this was before my time, when he was the officer in charge." Michael pushed for Rapid's parent company to cover his debts, but the IRS held him personally liable.

Kachroo may have fancied herself a business ace, but she appears to have met her match in Candace and Michael. One clue she'd been outflanked came, perhaps, at a dinner Candace had scheduled for Rapid's management and select investors the third week of September. Though Candace had died a week before, the group still convened, in part because she'd invited MerriBeth Adams, the CEO of Candace and Michael's previous company, AITI, which had been funded by Eckart Wintzen. Adams was an expert in FDA regulations and protocols, and Candace had led Kachroo to believe she had clinical study data that was relevant to Rapid. However, Kachroo, Evan, Mark Lloyd-Fox, and Vivian Komori now suspect this dinner was meant to be Candace's "big reveal." She'd intended to confess her wrongdoing, they say, as well as Michael's complicity with Laznicka.

But what, exactly, had Candace done wrong, and why include MerriBeth Adams?

As Rapid's investors would later learn, upon joining forces with Laznicka and then with Kachroo, Candace and Michael had omitted a detail crucial to their business: when AITI filed for bankruptcy, Eckart Wintzen had relinquished the exclusive patent license for Peptide T to Adams, who had placed the assets into a separate company, Peptide T Holdings (PTH), with plans to work with Jeff Galpin, the infectious disease specialist who had applied for a provisional patent on Peptide T to study its effect on PML a decade before. This meant that Rapid had been launched on a lie, as Candace and Michael had no legal right to develop the drugs they claimed to own.

"At that dinner, my mom wanted to let everyone know that Merri-Beth had the rights, and she wanted to work out a deal to bring Merri-Beth into the company so they could legitimately work on Peptide T," Evan says. "She was planning to come clean."

"Eckart chose [Adams] over us," Michael now admits, explaining that he and Candace had tried to work with Adams previously, hoping to procure a sublicense to develop Peptide T solely as a treatment for HIV. But Adams had demanded $200,000, which the couple could never afford. "She had the license rights and we found out she wasn't employed, so we said, 'Let's bury the hatchet on everything that happened before. You consult and work for us in the new company, and let's see if we can rescue some of this stuff,'" Michael continues. "She still had all the records, so we introduced her to Gaytri and brought her in."

After a tumultuous tenure at AITI, Adams had no desire to support Candace and Michael, but she saw a capable partner in Kachroo, and she knew that Rapid AG was hamstrung without her. Plus, she later claimed that Michael had said Rapid's management was aware of the licensing problem and encouraged her to "let sleeping dogs lie." Without funding of her own, Adams also lacked a game plan to monetize her intellectual property, so she never raised the specific issue of patent infringements with Kachroo. As a result, Kachroo assumed that the purpose of meeting Adams was to acquire clinical study information and rights to pursue Peptide T/DAPTA as a cure for PML.

During the fall of 2013 Kachroo engaged Adams as a consultant to Rapid's management, and on December 20 the women, along with Galpin, finalized a "Data Transfer Agreement" to acquire all data and IP from AITI, PTH, and related entities. In exchange, Adams and Galpin were to receive consulting and/or employment agreements and positions as FDA regulatory affairs officer and chief medical or clinical development officer, as well as no less than 1 percent of Rapid AG shares each, subject to current shareholders' approval of a stock option plan.

However, Adams wanted more assurance up front, preferably in the form of cash, so in June 2014 Kachroo amended the Data Transfer Agreement, assessing the value of rights and data reassigned at $750,000, which Rapid AG was to pay to Adams with either cash, company shares at a nominal value of $125.74 per share, or a combination of both. In her December 2014 CEO's update Kachroo announced to shareholders that Rapid AG "had acquired all intellectual property and clinical data emanating from AITI and Peptide T Holdings" and asserted that this acquisition "ensures that the intellectual property of the company remains unencumbered."

However, in January 2015 at the J. P. Morgan Healthcare Conference in San Francisco, Kachroo received a startling jolt. She'd organized a meeting with seven executives from a large pharmaceutical company she hoped would purchase part of Rapid. Instead, she learned that their due diligence had unearthed damning information: Candace and Michael were forbidden from commercializing Peptide T.

After the couple had been banished from the NIH for disseminating Peptide T underground and using federal government labs to launch a commercial venture, the NIH had agreed not to prosecute on the condition that Candace and Michael leave quietly. Because the NIH held the patent for Peptide T, officials assumed the couple would never be granted a license. Clearly, the Office of Technology Transfer had blocked access at every turn.

If Candace and Michael were prohibited from working on Peptide T, then how had they possibly come this far in three separate companies? It all came back to their nonprofit Integra Institute. By nabbing the European patent rights and establishing Integra, their lawyer had found a workaround, at least when it came to their first company, Peptide Design. By its very nature, a nonprofit could not be accused of trying to commercialize Peptide T. However, when Candace and Michael lost Bristol-Myers's backing, the NIH Office of Technology Transfer was wise to the couple's ploy and split their license as a result, effectively cutting them off at the knees.

Though Candace and Michael had claimed to own Peptide T and its analogues when they began working with Eckart Wintzen in 1990, he soon discovered that their license through Peptide Design had been suspended due to nonpayment of fees and a failure to meet milestones. Wintzen spent millions to procure an exclusive license, but when Merri-Beth Adams joined AITI in 1995, she was summoned to the NIH's Office of Technology Transfer and informed that AITI's license was being revoked again, in part because Candace and Michael had meddled in the NIMH's Phase II study led by Ellen Stover.

Wintzen and Adams managed to rectify all noncompliance, and they assured the government that Candace and Michael would play no future management roles within their firm. The couple was relegated to consultant status, and within two years AITI had procured exclusive licenses to develop Peptide T and its analogues for HIV, psoriasis, neuropsychiatric deficits including autism, and chronic fatigue syndrome.

Regardless, according to both Adams's affidavit and a subsequent investigation by the law firm DLA Piper, in August 2004, while still working for AITI, Candace and Michael had incorporated Rapid Pharmaceuticals and continued to perform research and development on Peptide T without a license, using proprietary data stolen from their previous employer. This violated both their employment and termination agreements, as the latter stipulated that they were required to return all proprietary data and information belonging to AITI. In their termination agreement, the couple was reminded of their noncompete and confidentiality commitments and was forbidden from working on Peptide T (i.e., "Immediately upon receipt of notice of termination, the Investigators shall stop the Research").

Worse, in 2006, while Adams was finalizing her exclusive license for PTH, she discovered that in December 2005, Candace and Michael had executed a feasibility study agreement with Aegis Therapeutics, LLC, a venture-backed company in San Diego that owned technology to stabilize peptides for oral consumption. With flagrant disregard for the law and in breach of their agreements with AITI/PTH, Candace and Michael planned to combine Aegis intellectual property with compounds they purported to own and have rights to, in order to create an oral version of Peptide T. As a result, Candace and Michael were hauled into the NIH Office of Technology Transfer and reprimanded for infringing on NIH patent rights as well as AITI/PTH's licenses.

This meant that DAPTA, the more stable version of Peptide T, which Candace and Michael had developed and patented at Georgetown after their termination, had been created illegally and was the property of AITI/PTH. Shockingly, based on DLA Piper's review of United States Patent and Trademark Office filings, Candace and Michael still proceeded to file process patent applications for this compound (renamed RAP-101) and even filed an application that contained proprietary information belonging to Aegis Therapeutics.

By the time Laznicka arrived to launch Rapid AG, the couple assumed that no one would remember the terms of their ignominious departure from the NIH twenty years prior. And because Eckart Wintzen died in 2008, they knew that MerriBeth Adams lacked financial means to fight them. "They assumed they could keep it a secret from the NIH," Evan says. "Would the patent office ever find out? Probably not. How would the NIH have found out unless someone told them?"

Rapid AG did not hold any valid title or assets, yet Candace and Michael proceeded to recruit unwitting investors, raising millions of dollars on intellectual property they did not own and were forbidden from monetizing. Perhaps by developing DAPTA, the couple fooled themselves and others into believing that they were working on a different substance, one that would be exempt from their obligations to AITI/PTH. But their feasibility study agreement with Aegis even lists the compound in question as "peptide T (DAPTA) and analogs," and Rapid's final chief scientific officer, Robert Fremeau, refers to it similarly in an affidavit. "RAP-101 (DAPTA) is a peptide that was discovered first in 1986," he writes. "It was patented thereafter, but the composition of matter patent has expired." Despite any claims to the contrary, Candace and Michael had been working on Peptide T all along, and Rapid AG was a house of cards.

"Candace and Michael believed that if they could get this drug as far along as possible, their many sins would be washed away," explains Mark Lloyd-Fox. "Candace did invent everything she claimed, but she wasn't the rightful owner; by contracts the title belonged to her employer. She and Michael didn't have the license. If I'm driving your car, just because I've got the keys and the vehicle, it doesn't mean I own it. I can't sell it to you."

In 2015, when Gaytri Kachroo assembled the pharmaceutical executives, she was hoping for a windfall. Instead she learned that her company was a worthless shell. Upon leaving the office suite, she and Michael walked all over San Francisco fighting. When he finally confessed to lying about the license, Kachroo called Evan in a frantic state, interrogating him about what he knew and when he'd come to know it. "She found out it was a sham," Evan says. "She'd put her career on the line with this pharma company, and they'd done their research."

Candace may have been desperate to get Peptide T to the masses, but Evan also believes that the moment his mother and Michael got a taste of wealth, they were hooked. They'd embarked on a spending spree in the wake of Peptide Design, and when the firm collapsed they'd found themselves in over their heads financially. "My mom used to tell me that we were going to have $100 million. She'd say, 'How long do you think before I'm recognized in the street?'" he says. "I remember when they got the new house. They were doing a lot of work on it and that cost a lot of money. Then they bought a boat for $105,000." The couple had also helped purchase apartments for Mildred and Wynne at a luxury complex in Bethesda, as well as a condominium in Los Angeles for Brandon, and were funding lavish vacations for Candace's extended family.

Reflecting on Candace's complicity, Evan still wonders how much his mother knew. "She didn't want to know. In her childish way, she would rationalize: 'We're not robbing people. We'll get them all the money back because it's going to be great,'" he says. "She had an idea that if she could claim ignorance, if she didn't know the whole truth, then somehow she wasn't guilty. Michael knew, but since Laznicka was benefitting him with money and these trips to Switzerland to see his girlfriend, he was turning a blind eye too."

Investors say that Candace did know, for Laznicka had discovered the couple's lie and was holding it over their heads. In January 2008, after receiving a statement from the couple's attorneys at Greenberg Traurig reiterating that Candace and Michael held no assets, Laznicka had accompanied them to the NIH's Office of Technology Transfer to seek a license. Of course, they were denied because the exclusive license belonged to MerriBeth Adams. Laznicka then approached Adams independently, but she turned him down. At this point, Kachroo and investors say, he ceased to contribute his own money but continued to solicit funds from others. "He was furious and swearing at them in emails, and Candace was saying she's sorry," Lloyd-Fox says. "With full knowledge of this, Pert, Ruff, and Laznicka went out to take our money and secure us as founders."

Kachroo, Mark Lloyd-Fox, and Vivian Komori also claim that the couple falsified documents to the FDA and Whitman-Walker Clinic. Obviously, it is illegal to manufacture and distribute a drug without FDA authorization or the rights to underlying intellectual property. Because Rapid's management team lacked fundamental assets, they were unable to contract with an approved laboratory that met safety standards for the Whitman-Walker trial. A legitimate lab would have been obliged to check the composition-of-matter patent before proceeding. So to avoid being exposed, Candace and Michael misled Whitman-Walker officials and illicitly made Peptide T at Rapid Labs. Moreover, Gaytri Kachroo discerned that the couple had supported

Laznicka's black market all along. "Candace and Mike confessed to me that they were distributing Peptide T," she says.

In early 2015, shortly after Kachroo discovered Candace and Michael's deceit, Jeff Galpin was surprised when she and Adams approached to ask him to place Rapid AG's patent licenses in his name. The women didn't mention the license dispute, but still, this sounded fishy. Galpin understood the need for a doctor or scientist to lend scientific legitimacy that Kachroo and Adams lacked as pure businesspeople, but why not put the licenses in Michael's name? He guessed it was because, after twenty years, Candace and Michael had failed to show significant results and the NIH Office of Technology Transfer had turned them down. And, given Candace and Michael's reputations, he also suspected foul play.

"I spent a lot of my time warning MerriBeth to get out of there. I told her to quit. She was still getting some payment that she needed for her family. She was desperate for money. She didn't beg, but she came close, as did Gaytri," says Galpin. "Gaytri wanted me and MerriBeth to do something that would have been incredibly dangerous legally. She tried to ensnare us to take responsibility for something we didn't even know was legally available. I said, 'No, thank you. It ain't worth the heartburn.' They thought I was going to be swayed by talking to the Kennedy family in Boston. Maybe I was a chicken or maybe I felt like playing doctor and not lawyer or Perry Mason for the rest of my life. I felt like I'd be the fall guy at the end of the show."

Unable to sway Galpin, Kachroo flew around the globe informing Rapid's shareholders of the couple's alleged IP fraud. Initially she was stunned when some didn't seem fazed—until she realized that they already knew! Many were wealthy HIV-positive men who understood that Rapid was a ruse and, in fact, had been paying not for a stake in the company but rather to receive Peptide T. This explained how Laznicka had been able to raise $8.85 million without diluting his stake: he'd structured most contributions as loans rather than equity positions. In so doing, he wasn't beholden to disclose the inner workings of management and had protected his "investors" from Rapid's wrongs. He was also free to "skim the cream."

Had Michael and Laznicka purposely racked up debt and failed to pay taxes because they intended to run Rapid into the ground? Kachroo didn't want a bankruptcy on her record, but she understood that if the company went belly-up, they'd have waltzed away with investors' money and their debts would be forgiven. Perhaps this had been their plan all along.

Candace, however, had a conscience. She knew that the inquiry Mark Lloyd-Fox had ordered would reveal her and Michael's transgressions, and it weighed heavily on her. Just a month before she died, her aunt Lillian passed away after a prolonged battle with Alzheimer's disease. When Candace arrived in Florida for the funeral, she began wailing at the gravesite, as though for the death of a child rather than an elderly aunt who'd been declining for years. Throughout her visit, she asked family members, "What do you think if I wear blue and white stripes? How will I look in stripes?" This made no sense at the time, as no one knew then that Candace feared going to jail.

"It was killing Candace that I'd sold my apartment in Covent Garden to invest in Rapid. When Laznicka couldn't make payroll in 2010, she knew I gave him $100,000," Lloyd-Fox says. "It was killing her, and she was urging me not to do things that she knew she needed. It was like a mother looking after her own, yet I didn't know the full story behind it. The more generous and giving I became, the more she was conflicted. She was desperate to tell me stuff. She'd go a little way down there and then stop short. She became increasingly uncomfortable with what she knew to be the truth."

Similarly, the week before Candace died, in preparation for the dinner she'd organized with MerriBeth Adams, Candace promised Kachroo that she'd "soon know everything and was sure [Kachroo] could fix it." "Candace may have been crazy, but she was brilliant and passionate. She had real heart and empathy," Kachroo says. "She didn't want their lie to stand. She wanted me to be CEO of a real company with real IP."

Though Kachroo and Michael seemed intent on working together in the wake of Candace's death, the moment Kachroo unearthed the couple's shameful backstory, she mobilized with Adams to expel Michael from the company. On January 29, 2015, she changed the locks at Rapid Labs and seized all records, computers, notebooks, and data, which she had transported to a storage facility in Cambridge, Massachusetts, as well as drug compounds related to Rapid AG's patent licenses. On March 15 Kachroo wrote to Rapid's board announcing an investigation into Michael's "alleged IP related fraud," and the following day she filed criminal trespass charges against him for entering the Maryland laboratories, though these were dismissed after two weeks.

According to the minutes of a Rapid board meeting on March 23, Kachroo alerted federal authorities and, along with Adams, visited the Maryland state attorney's office to file criminal charges against Michael. Kachroo states that Adams had wanted to sanction Candace and Michael previously for infringing upon AITI/PTH's licenses, but she feared that the couple's shareholders would fight her. However, now that the cat was out of the bag, Adams threatened to rescind her Data Transfer Agreement, and Kachroo advocated to reassign any assets Rapid could procure into a new company that would establish a chain of title for all patent licenses, free and clear.

On April 5, Kachroo sent a letter to Rapid shareholders claiming that the board had concluded that "there is no way to raise further funds in Rapid because of legal and ethical violations Pre-2012 relating to IP assets and clinical development. Due to the over-indebtedness of the Company as of today, the Board was forced to decide to liquidate the current enterprise without delay." The following month, Rapid's accountants and auditor at KPMG warned that the company was overindebted by at least CHF 3.9 million and might be required to file for bankruptcy.

A battle for Rapid ensued, as Kachroo and Michael embarked on competing lawsuits. During their three years of mudslinging, Michael claims that Kachroo filed reports with the FBI and informed the Montgomery County Police that he'd killed his wife. Kachroo made an unsuccessful bid to launch Arise BioPharma, a new company she hoped would provide a clean title to AITI/PTH's intellectual property unencumbered by Rapid AG's contingent liabilities. However, she was stymied after Cynthia Ingraham, the London client who'd funded Rapid's autism studies, pursued her for failure to disclose conflict of interest, overcharging, and misusing funds. For this, among other charges, Kachroo received a three-year suspension from the Massachusetts bar in 2018, and subsequently from the New York bar in 2020. By that time, Kachroo's beloved mother was dying, and she was too drained to appeal.

Once Ingraham turned against Kachroo, investors say she grew claws, throwing her full weight behind Michael and funding his case to bury their mutual enemy Kachroo. This he was more than happy to do—even if it meant enlisting the help of his former foe Laznicka. Ironically, Michael's duel with Kachroo reunited him with Laznicka, whom he was suddenly quick to forgive, and with support from Stephen Kennedy Smith, the men moved to elect a new board of advisors.

"Laznicka isn't a crook at all," Michael now insists, contradicting earlier statements. "I would say he's a smooth operator. I don't think he's a fraud or lied or broke any contracts with us. Maybe we just weren't aligned on the direction of the company. Laznicka's out there and, at the end of the day, he did organize against Gaytri, which helped me out. He joined with me to have the controlling vote to kick her out of the company. So we'll make nice and gloss over the other stuff." By joining forces against Kachroo at the end, Michael and Laznicka shrewdly shielded themselves.

Rapid AG filed for bankruptcy in February 2016, and for a time investors contemplated suing the company's leadership team. But a lawsuit seemed costly and even the shareholders with resources to fight were too exhausted and overwhelmed to proceed. Instead, they decided to cut their losses. According to Lloyd-Fox and Komori, Laznicka invited the Rapid shareholders who'd sided with him to roll the value of their Rapid shares into a new venture, San Diego–based Vault Pharma, Inc., for which he went on to raise additional money.

In 2016, Laznicka was interviewed by the *Los Angeles Business Journal* for a series on immigrant entrepreneurs, and when asked when and why he arrived in the United States, he made no mention of Rapid AG. Instead he claimed that in 2011 California governor Gray Davis introduced him to UCLA "for potential partnerships in biological sciences" and that he'd decided to stay because of the compelling opportunity "to make a massive global impact in health management for cancer and vaccines."

Seven years later, Rapid's employees and shareholders are still licking their wounds. Padma Oza says that she worked for six months without a salary and when Rapid declared bankruptcy she was paid only $12,000 of the $23,000 she was owed. Mark Lloyd-Fox moved to South Africa and, on the advice of his clinicians, has gone back on ARVs. The last time he checked, $300,000 worth of Peptide T was sitting in a freezer in Rockville, Maryland, but he can't get access to it. "There's nothing the ARVs are giving me right now that will diminish everything Peptide T has done," he says. "But now we'll never know. We'll never know how Peptide T could have helped others."

Lloyd-Fox lost not only his money but also the trust of many wealthy associates he'd convinced to invest. The experience at Rapid was, he says, as ruinous as receiving his HIV diagnosis. For sixteen years he has been in recovery for alcohol and drugs, and he estimates that during that time he's had 120 days of relapse on alcohol, in part because of the Rapid fiasco. "The cost to Vivian, myself, and others has been enormous—years of hell, thinking you know one thing, finding out another," he says. "At one point, I was absolutely destitute. It was the most challenging and distressing period of my life."

Candace and Michael didn't repay Vivian Komori within a year, as promised; in fact, they didn't reimburse her at all, even though they were raking in combined salaries of $270,000 at Rapid. Komori's husband was forced to take a second job selling produce, and it wasn't until fifteen years later, when she received an inheritance after her mother's death, that the couple was finally able to pay off their loan.

"It's gut-wrenching, heartbreaking, and unconscionable, what they did. You might think you get away with stuff, that you've lined your own pocketbook, but you're not going to get away with it forever. I have to believe they'll be brought to justice," Komori says, fighting back tears. "I still had full faith in Candace. I think she really meant well and believed they would be able to get all this done, and everything would be hunky-dory. She was sick, so I didn't hold it against her even after I found out they screwed us. I can't say that about Michael Ruff. Michael Ruff is all about the money, all the way through. The $250,000 was a huge sacrifice for us. He knew that, readily took it, and crapped all over us. What kind of person does that?

"Prior to all of this, I always thought the best of people—that they're good at heart," she continues. "But there are people who don't care who they hurt if you get in their way. This whole experience changed me for the rest of my life. I will never be the same."

As for Jeff Galpin, he knows he dodged a bullet by walking away from the mess that is Peptide T, and the hubris that destroyed its creators. Still, he mourns the loss of a drug that had the potential to heal. "There's a moral to be taught in all of this—not only the loss of a good idea, taking something good and prostituting it, but also what research should be. It should be honest, not throwing people under the bus for ill-gotten gains. Who knows who [Peptide T] might have saved if given the right set of studies conducted appropriately? This is the tragedy of a drug that never had its day, that never had a chance to be right."

CHAPTER SIXTEEN

RELEASE THE SPIRIT

THOUGH CANDACE CAST HER WORK AS A SPIRITUAL QUEST, SHE LABORED TO SURmount a thirst for recognition and revenge, and ultimately remained hostage to her ego. Despite her public pledge to a higher power, she engaged in behavior that was both immoral and illegal, behaving as though she were beyond reproach. But it's important to remember that she wasn't acting in a vacuum.

At Hopkins, Candace was groomed to be ruthless in a world of callous competition. At the NIH, she operated within a culture of pervasive venality that rewarded men like Bob Gallo. And there seemed to be no stopping what Dr. Drummond Rennie, deputy editor of the *Journal of the American Medical Association*, called Big Pharma's "race to the ethical bottom." Time and again, Candace was steeped in enmity, then outfoxed and brought to her knees. All of this happened in the name of healing and was, after all, how the game was played.

A game is defined by its rules, agreed upon by players. So one can't help but wonder what happens when rules are discarded and standards break down. What happens when the institutions charged with protecting public health are, to their very core, rank with sickness? What turns a good woman bad?

In light of Rapid's internecine battles and Candace's vow to come clean, her family and friends found the timing of her death uncanny. Naturally, one wonders if the cause was confirmed by an autopsy. "No, no autopsy," Michael says, explaining that in Maryland, an investigation is not mandated if someone has died at home alone. Candace had been having trouble breathing for a week before she died and her lips appeared blue, he recounts. So, given her family's history of aneurysms and strokes, Michael assumed she'd developed a blood clot that lodged in her heart. Thus his decision to announce that Candace succumbed to cardiac arrest in September 2013.

As Michael tells it, the morning of Candace's death, he went into the office to work with Rapid's administrator Padma Oza on the company's taxes while Candace worked from home. They'd been on a phone call and were due to begin another, but when Michael called Candace, she didn't pick up. He became worried and drove home, only to find her dead in the bushes outside. Michael imagines that Candace had been sitting with her coffee and her laptop on the back deck and had gotten up to walk toward the pool, where she liked to sunbathe nude. She'd likely collapsed en route.

No forensics investigation was ever performed; EMTs simply arrived at the house and took Candace's body straight to the hospital. While her time of death was unconfirmed, it feels to Candace's children curiously close to the moment she wrote her final email in support of Kachroo. The email was sent at 12:43 p.m. and, according to Padma Oza, Michael left the office shortly after receiving it. It would have taken him ten minutes to drive home, and Evan and Vanessa say that he called them at around 1:25 p.m. to report that their mother was dead.

Candace's family and friends suspect that hormone treatments may have played a role. They know that, a year before her death, Candace had begun the Wiley Protocol, a controversial hormone replacement technique meant to mimic a woman's natural twenty-eight-day cycle that has been criticized by the medical community for its side effects and lack of empirical evidence. Candace was also ordering supplemental estrogen from China online, and she'd bragged to friends about her renewed youth and vigor. Disturbingly, she had begun menstruating again at age sixty-seven and stashing her used, bloody tampons under candles and rocks around her backyard swimming pool.

For the sake of Candace's legacy and the future of Rapid, no one wanted talk of bloody tampons around the pool. But many questioned whether her elevated hormones had created a clot that caused heart failure. It certainly seemed to have exacerbated her mania. The week before she died, Candace met her daughter, Vanessa, who until recently was a branch chief at the Federal Emergency Management Agency, at Mears Marina in Annapolis, where Candace and Michael kept their boat. As they were leaving, Candace became agitated in the parking lot and told Vanessa that Michael was having yet another affair and wanted a divorce, and that he'd made her change her will, but that Candace was planning to change it back. "My mom made it sound like Michael didn't love her, that he was after money, notoriety, research," Vanessa recalls. "She was very distraught."

Candace's general practitioner, Zidi Berger, says she was never informed of supplemental estrogen, nor had she learned until the night before Candace died that she had been having trouble breathing. "I was so upset, I can't even tell you, when I heard that. She was not sick. She didn't have any illness. She was a very healthy person, just overweight and stressed," Berger says, noting that just six months prior, Candace had gone hiking at high altitudes in Peru.

Berger was at the airport that evening, preparing to depart for a conference abroad, when she received a call from Michael, who described Candace's symptoms. Fearing that Candace was having a pulmonary embolism, Berger called Sibley Memorial Hospital in Arlington, Virginia, to secure a bed in the emergency room and told Michael to rush his wife there at once. She had to board her flight then and couldn't follow up, so Berger learned days later that Candace never made it. "There is intervention for a pulmonary embolism. They get you in the ICU and give you drugs, and they get you back to normal," she says. "It used to kill people, but now they treat it like a stroke. People can survive, but you have to go to a hospital!"

Candace's family acknowledges that she would have resisted going to the hospital, as she equated it with being institutionalized. But they cannot understand why Michael didn't call an ambulance, or at least summon Evan to intervene, as he had done every other time Candace grew problematic.

The day of Candace's death, Michael seemed stoic when he phoned Evan, yet when Vanessa arrived two hours later at Adventist Health-Care Shady Grove Hospital in Rockville, where Candace's body was taken, she found her stepfather wailing and throwing medical equipment around the room. As Michael was erupting, a hospital worker entered to ask whether he wanted an autopsy performed and Michael declined. When Vanessa pushed back, Michael spoke in graphic terms, insisting that Candace "would never want to be carved up. She wouldn't want her brain all sliced up." Evan also lobbied to reconsider, arguing that Candace's genetic offspring should know if she had an underlying medical condition they might inherit.

Michael's subsequent behavior seemed crass and insensitive to friends and family as well. In an email about Candace's memorial service that Michael sent to friends ten days after her death, his tone sounds enthusiastic and promotional. "I have a comment re: [New York Times], which did a wonderful obit (like below), but wait, there's more!" he writes, before proceeding to criticize the newspaper for drawing too much attention to Candace's initial discoveries while failing to publicize her more recent efforts to treat HIV, Alzheimer's, and chronic pain. In response, Michael spends the next three paragraphs of his email promoting their collaborative work and his business.

Additionally, Michael directed the Baltimore crematorium to Evan to confirm his mother's identity, and he and his sisters wasted no time sifting through Candace's belongings and throwing them away. He disposed of Candace's collection of books signed by luminaries and refused to give her children family photos and heirlooms, even when items were of little value. Eventually Michael relinquished Candace's pottery and some of her jewelry, but only after he'd catalogued it to ensure that nothing was of value. Before long, however, Michael showed up at Vanessa's door to ask for the jewelry back.

"He didn't want her kids in the house after her death. He has this very strange way of talking: 'Damn kids! They want to come in and rifle through her stuff and I'm the husband. It's my stuff. It's my house.' He was saying it in his matter-of-fact, sarcastic way—not compassionate at all," Lydia Temoshok says. "It didn't even occur to him that the children should be speaking at Candace's memorial service. His emotional reactions were so far off from what a husband's would be like."

Michael's conduct in other areas of life proved unsettling to family and friends as well. Within days of Candace's death he told Vanessa that he was eager to date and would likely be married in a year. "He said, 'Do you think if I find a younger woman, I can still have children?'" she recalls. And before Mark Lloyd-Fox became aware of Michael's role in Rapid's scandals, Michael requested a meeting with his mother, Ann Keen, the British MP, who was visiting Washington,

D.C. Keen assumed it was business-related, but during lunch Michael put his hand on her knee and suggested that they "console and comfort each other" now that their spouses were both dead. He then invited Keen back to his house. "[My mother] said, 'I don't know how to tell you this, but I was actually disgusted,'" Lloyd-Fox says. "She paid the bill herself and walked away. She said, 'I have never, ever been propositioned this way.'"

Weeks after Candace's death, Michael bragged to Adam "Omkara" Helfer, a spiritual healer who'd been a close friend and advisor to Candace, that he could "go one of two ways, and both of these women had spoken at Candace's memorial"; presumably this meant that Michael planned to pursue either Gaytri Kachroo or Gilah Rosner, a horticulturist and home chef who'd been preparing Candace's meals. To Helfer, this seemed distastefully soon, and he felt perplexed by both options, particularly Rosner.

During the disastrous year before she died, Candace had been dazed and fragile as her marriage collapsed and her dreams were shattered. While Michael was in Switzerland on one of his many jaunts, she'd sought solace at Sanctuary, a twenty-eight-acre spiritual retreat center in rural Beallsville, Maryland, where Gilah (née Gayle Lauren) Rosner worked as a manager. When Candace arrived, Rosner was starstruck. As a PhD chemist who'd spent many years working in labs, she recognized Candace and saw in her a kindred spirit who also operated at the junction of science and spirituality.

Though Rosner had earned her doctorate studying experimental pathology and performed clinical fellowships in hematology, immunopathology, and molecular genetics, she'd abandoned her scientific career to embark on a spiritual path after her parents had died of cancer just ten weeks apart. Rosner now devoted herself to Kabbalah and lived in a modest apartment on Sanctuary's grounds. It was here that

Candace unburdened herself to this fellow scientist and seeker, blaming her snowballing weight on stress. Soon after, Rosner began advising Candace on nutrition and health.

Following Candace's death, however, her inner circle was stunned when Rosner commandeered the memorial service, portraying herself as Candace's heir apparent. None of them had ever heard of Rosner, yet here she was claiming to be Candace's best friend. Indeed, in a Facebook post four days after Candace's death, Rosner announced that "[Candace] called me her 'angel' and now it is up to me to see myself through her eyes," and she continues to maintain that Candace "brought me in to finish the job. I got elected by her to finish the job."

Those closest to Candace consider this nothing short of preposterous. Though Michael and Rosner deny it, the reigning suspicion is that they were having an affair. Candace deduced this as well; months before she died, she called Nancy Morris crying because Michael had taken Rosner out on the couple's boat alone. She also told Mark Lloyd-Fox that she thought her husband was betraying her with a new "friend."

Before long, her family grew uneasy as Michael seemed increasingly influenced by this woman. The evening of Candace's memorial, when about forty close friends and family members gathered at her home for a reception, Michael and Rosner stunned guests when they took down the five-by-six-foot photo of Candace's smiling face that had hung near the altar to a Buddha statue in the back garden. Then Michael smashed the picture, poured lighter fluid on it, and burned it ritualistically, telling family members that it was Rosner's plan to "release the spirit."

Three months later, at a family Christmas party, Michael announced that he and Rosner were a couple, and by the following March she had moved into Candace's house. On the one-year anniversary of Candace's death, Michael and Rosner used the occasion to host a fundraiser for Sanctuary, where they charged an entrance fee and handed out brochures promoting Rapid Pharmaceuticals. It wasn't long before Rosner left Sanctuary to work with Michael on his latest venture, Creative Bio-Peptides—cleverly named to evoke Candace Beebe Pert—and leveraged Candace's Rolodex to align herself with Joan Borysenko, the pioneer in integrative health with whom Rosner now organizes spiritual and culinary retreats. Like so many others, Rosner has profited from her brief association with Candace.

Making matters worse, to fund his legal battle with Kachroo, Michael forced the sale of the Los Angeles apartment Candace had purchased for her younger son, Brandon, though he acknowledged that Candace never would have agreed. And after waiting a year to arrange for Candace's interment at the Beebe family plot in Lyme, Connecticut, Michael dithered over the cost of a tombstone. Instead of having a gravesite prepared professionally, he enlisted Evan to dig the hole for his mother's ashes. "What son has to dig his own mother's grave?" Vanessa asks through tears.

At that point, Candace's children were still trying to maintain a relationship with their stepfather; he'd always been awkward, they say, but they didn't want to believe he was evil. Yet when Michael's conduct became too distressing to ignore, Candace's children demanded to see her will and trust. Despite Candace's warning to Vanessa the week before she died, they had never laid eyes on her will, much less attempted to contest it, because they assumed Michael would make good on her wishes. Plus Candace had been manic for some time, so her children assumed that she was delusional or crying wolf, particularly regarding her will. She'd even gathered the family a year prior in a restaurant in Annapolis to discuss their inheritance. Candace had said she'd put aside $1 million, and in the event of her death Evan would be the executor assigned to distribute gifts to the siblings, as well as her sister Deane and Deane's children. At the time Candace and Michael were drawing up contracts with Gaytri Kachroo for a new company in which her children would own a combined 5 percent. Candace was anticipating a financial bonanza then and assuring her children that they'd all be millionaires. Why would she ever excise them from her will?

However, when Candace's children got hold of it, they found it in contradiction with her expressed wishes; Michael was now the recipient of all assets and they had been entirely cut out. Immediately Evan consulted a top lawyer in Washington, D.C., who said that Candace's signatures were valid even though she was mentally ill. But her children believe that this represents Michael's desires, not their mother's, and that he manipulated a sick woman into authorizing a document that served only him. Regardless, by the time Candace's family realized that Michael was up to no good, they had missed their window to contest the will; according to Maryland law, Evan says, they would have had to challenge Michael within a year of their mother's death.

Candace's family also grew perturbed by the visceral nature of Michael and Rosner's enmity toward Gaytri Kachroo. After the meeting in San Francisco in January 2015 at which Kachroo uncovered Michael's alleged patent fraud, she became "public enemy number one." According to Evan and Nancy Kingcaid, Michael and Rosner then printed memes of Kachroo (e.g., her face on a gorilla, her face on someone in an orange jumpsuit in jail) and hung them up around the house. Rosner also fabricated a burlap voodoo doll stuffed with apothecary plants on which she pinned a swatch of fabric from a scarf Kachroo had left behind. She then stuck pins in the doll, "wishing [Kachroo] to fall down the stairs and break her neck," Kingcaid says. "They were really graphic about it."

In an April 2015 email to family, Michael writes that it's "time to burn the voodoo doll (it exists) in a modest, v modest I'd say, ceremony, with lighter fluid. Which will end with me pissing it out. Send your samples, well packed, I'll toss them on for good measure too." Later, in July 2019, he comments casually during a phone interview that "Gaytri had a voodoo doll, so we thought we should have a voodoo doll," as though this were commonplace. After being chastised by Rosner, however, he swears never to speak of it again.

Eventually Evan launched an investigation into all aspects of his mother's death. Though it is not unusual for grieving family members to lay blame after an untimely passing, some found his resolve extreme. After an exhaustive survey of Michael's comportment and correspondence, he delivered a binder of evidence he'd collected to the police in Rockville, who remain stumped by a lack of physical evidence. "The detective said, 'In Maryland, no body, no crime.' Without an autopsy, they couldn't do an investigation," Evan says. "No one would do an investigation. They said we'd waited too long, but in the moment, we were in shock. Even if we were suspicious, it was so quick, we had no time."

If outsiders were quick to discount Evan, it was because he too had begun to show signs of bipolar disorder. He'd been gifted with his mother's scientific brilliance and, from a young age, had served as Candace's sparring partner and sounding board. He'd studied electrical engineering at the University of Michigan and worked in technology jobs in California before returning to Maryland to pursue a master's degree. Up until his mother's death, Evan was always garrulous and enthusiastic, and his high energy manifested as passion rather than mania. When Candace died, however, his explorations took a morbid turn.

The more Evan researched, the more he became convinced that Candace did not die of natural causes. Solving the mystery of his mother's death proved an obsession, and soon it became clear that Evan had inherited not only Candace's sharp mind but also her mental illness. Though it is rare to exhibit signs of bipolar disorder so late in life, the stress Evan weathered in his late forties drove him over the edge.

When Evan discovered that he and his siblings had been cut from Candace's will and that Michael had reunited with "the viper" Laznicka against Kachroo, he began sending rambling emails with details of his stepfather's culpability. Those on the receiving end felt compassion and concern, but mostly they were overwhelmed. If Candace's life had seemed an exercise in finger-pointing and obfuscation, then Evan's antics after her death only compounded the drama. When Evan confided to Adam "Omkara" Helfer that he "might do something stupid," Michael filed a protective order and encouraged friends and family to cut ties with his stepson.

The more friends and family avoided Evan, the worse his condition grew. He had a series of manic breakdowns that began in March 2016, but he refused medication because, he says, "my mom had taught me not to take the pills." During the first half of 2018, he experienced mania so extreme that he quit his job as a primary patent examiner and was banned from the U.S. Patent and Trademark Office campus in Alexandria, Virginia, following an altercation with his supervisor, who'd advised him to seek counseling. In February 2019, Evan called Kingcaid for help and was hospitalized for two weeks, after which he improved dramatically. He is now freelancing as a patent agent in electrical engineering, and while he has a personal connection to the divine and pursues alternative treatments, he also takes mood-stabilizing medication.

A decade after their mother's death, Vanessa and Evan are still trying to process a harrowing series of events. "This destroyed my family. I couldn't handle it," Vanessa says. "Somehow, I compartmentalized, but I have to face what happened. It still feels as fresh. It's so traumatic for me. I deal with it every day." Indeed, in every conversation for this book she continues to ask, "Does Michael ever ask about us? Does he want to know how I'm doing?" And every time, the answer is no.

Candace's friends and colleagues also grapple with her premature passing, contemplating the wonders she might have accomplished had she lived. "Candace was a rebel. I don't know if people make fantastic discoveries that upend the world's view by conforming. Every genius disturbs society," says her friend Andrea Schara, the Bowen family systems therapist. "I used to say to Candace, 'It's worth it. Be different. Be yourself. To hell with the flak! Torpedoes ahead!' If you're living as a rebel, you already know you're representing a minority viewpoint that few people can hear. So, why not bring attention by becoming the glitter woman . . . like Candace was? No one's going to forget that. They might forget what you said, but they'll never forget who you are."

Candace was, without a doubt, unforgettable. She displayed a rich and striking duality, often appearing to be two people at once— an effusive, loving wunderkind breaking barriers to serve the greater good, and a raging egotist consumed by fear and fury, clamoring to be recognized and rewarded. Even with the best of intentions, she lacked sound judgment and was easily swayed, and her insecurity and desperation to be loved led to decisions that compromised not only her work but also her moral compass.

In the end, she was both a savior and a crook. When given choices, she often chose poorly, and her downfall was driven by internal and external forces alike. Yet perhaps, as Aristotle said, "no great mind has ever existed without a touch of madness." Instead of judging, one might acknowledge the blessing and burden of her unique skills and insight, and cradle Candace in the compassion she so seldom received in life. For Candace died as she'd always lived, in the eye of the storm.

EPILOGUE

"IF SOMEONE SAID, 'MICHAEL, HERE'S THE BOOK OF YOUR LIFE,' I WOULD HAVE read it and shot myself in the head," Michael says just before Thanksgiving 2019. "The trajectory of my life, the upward trajectory of my life? In some ways I'm still emerging from the shitstorm."

He continues to miss Candace, he says—her cheerleading and stubborn positivity, the way she made him believe. "I'd get depressed. I'd be moping and she'd say, 'It's already happened. You're already a success! Live out your destiny!'" Michael remembers. "She had such presence, a belief and confidence in how our life was going to play out. It was powerful and comforting."

Still, he forges ahead in his new firm, Creative Bio-Peptides, trying to commercialize a patent for RAP-103, the last compound Candace created before she died. Though Rapid AG alumni maintain that RAP-103 is yet another Peptide T derivative and thus the property of MerriBeth Adams and Peptide T Holdings, Michael paints it as a trump card. After all, he wants "$8 million in [his] bank account, not a half-million in [his] bank account," he says, and he appears to be on his way.

Somehow, NIH officials have forgotten or overlooked the couple's scandals and instead have opened their wallets. Despite misusing federal labs and being reproved multiple times by the NIH's Office of Technology Transfer for patent infringements, Michael has managed to secure more than $6 million in new grants from three separate NIH institutes.

Hypothesizing that RAP-103 blocks addiction, Michael received a $350,000 grant from the National Institute on Drug Abuse in April 2019. He was able to show that Candace's compound affects the opiate receptor to increase the potency of morphine, so less morphine is required to achieve desired results. This reduces both the motivation to take drugs and withdrawal symptoms. Because that program was a success and Michael's team met all milestones, he was awarded a second NIDA grant for $2.5 million in June 2021.

In September 2022, in the journal *Drug and Alcohol Dependence*, Creative Bio-Peptides announced findings from a preclinical study showing that treatment with RAP-103 lessened the severity of naloxone-precipitated withdrawal responses in morphine dependence, as well as morphine-induced respiratory depression. RAP-103 also normalized aspects of the brain that are altered by opioid abuse.

To be sure, creating a cure for opioid addiction would be a perfect conclusion to Candace's story. "When she found the opiate receptor, everyone thought they'd find the nonaddictive opiate—the holy grail, the sword in the stone," Michael says. "Instead, Candace found the drug that keeps you from wanting to be addicted. You have less pain and need less morphine, so you lower the abuse liability right there. She didn't live to see it, but it will work."

However, Michael sees inflammation-related disease as a far larger market and a faster route to his $8 million in the bank. Between 2020 and 2021 he was also awarded two separate $500,000 grants funded by the National Institute on Aging, based on the notion that—just as Jeff Galpin proposed years ago—Peptide T and its derivatives have implications for neurodegeneration.

Simultaneously, with scientific partners in Portugal, Michael is studying the dementia-like cognitive disorder that affects 80 percent of people afflicted with Parkinson's disease. "We're curing it in animals, so now we have a path to clinical trials for Parkinson's," he says. "I'm sure my drug's going to cure Alzheimer's and Parkinson's. Alzheimer's is loss of synapses. We make the synapses come back."

Separately, Michael secured a $3 million grant from the National Institute of Neurological Disorders and Stroke to test RAP-103 for diabetic neuropathic pain. "What happens in chronic pain is the same that happens with addictions. The neurons die," he says. "We can make chronic pain go away by reducing inflammation, and if you need to take opiates, you can take much less."

This grant, which took a while to be approved, was like "a slow hand job for four months," Michael says, and if he didn't receive it, he "was gonna call and say, 'I know where you live. I'm gonna throw snowballs through your window.'" Thankfully, that wasn't necessary, and this preclinical study was also successful. In July 2022, Creative Bio-Peptides announced in the journal *Life Sciences* that RAP-103 reduced the quantity of opioids needed after surgery by 50 percent and reversed chronic neuropathic pain caused by diabetes, which afflicts nearly half of all diabetics.

Michael has been so busy at Creative Bio-Peptides that he's hardly had time to pat himself on the back. But it feels good to be vindicated and acknowledged by his peers, and to emerge victorious after years of hardship. "[The NIH] is not giving me $6 million because I'm a good bullshitter. They're giving me $6 million because they think we've got a shot. It's all independent, peer-reviewed," he says. "It's going to be the culmination of Candy's life's work, my life's work.

"We were right in 1985. We just got beaten back because of limitations and the state of knowledge. But like a weed, we sprouted up in the playing field across the street," Michael continues. "By next year, the company could take the next big step to put this drug in clinical trials."

Michael wants what so many have desired—to profit from Candace's genius, following her beloved rainbow toward a pot of gold. Now that she's gone, will he succeed where others failed? "Candace was very intuitive; she could see around the corner," he says. "The story is: Candace launched an arrow, the arrow's in flight, and we're standing here saying, 'What's it gonna hit?'"

SOURCES

"Everyone likes to see a train wreck," Michael said as we embarked on interviews. "There are half a dozen wrecks in this story, a lot of villains, and a handful of heroes." Little did I know that separating villains from heroes would be my hardest task.

The tale I've unearthed is more twisted than I could have imagined, and few are who they seem. I began this process as a fangirl, in awe of Candace and wanting to believe the best of her, so I've often felt disappointed and duped as the extent of her and Michael's machinations became clear. Still, I want to thank Michael for being honest and forthcoming; in his words, he "spilled his guts" to me on matters both personal and professional, often against the advice of Gilah Rosner, who is now his wife. They and others may not like the resulting portrayal, but I hope they appreciate my duty to present an objective, journalistic report.

In the six years Michael and I have collaborated, I've repeated time and again that I aim to learn and tell the truth, just as Candace tried to do—at least in the end. In the face of conflicting viewpoints, particularly when Candace and Michael's version of events diverges from many others', I have done my best to present a balanced account. I have also worked to place the treachery I've uncovered in the context of broader systems that reward ruthless and dysfunctional behavior, for the true villain of this story is greed.

Introduction

Author's interview with Lisa Feldman Barrett, May 23, 2022.

Bessel A. van der Kolk, *The Body Keeps the Score: Brain, Mind, and Body in the Healing of Trauma* (New York: Penguin Books, 2014), 36–37.

Candace Pert, *Molecules of Emotion: Why You Feel the Way You Feel* (New York: Scribner, 1997), 271.

Lisa Feldman Barrett, *How Emotions Are Made: The Secret Life of the Brain* (New York: Houghton Mifflin Harcourt, 2017), 40, 66–67, 199–218.

Naomi Oreskes, *Why Trust Science?* (Princeton, NJ: Princeton University Press, 2019).

Chapter One: Eureka!

Author's interviews with Deborah Stokes, May 29, 2019; August 9, 2019; August 22, 2021.

Author's interviews with Edythe London, December 23, 2019; August 31, 2021; October 10, 2022.

Author's interviews with Agu Pert, July 9, 2019; March 18, 2022; July 1, 2022; July 9, 2022.

Candace Pert, *Molecules of Emotion: Why You Feel the Way You Feel* (New York: Scribner, 1997), 32–34, 37–40, 43–61.

Candace Pert, *Everything You Need to Know to Feel Go(o)d* (Carlsbad, CA: Hay House, 2006), 29–30.

Solomon H. Snyder, *Brainstorming: The Science and Politics of Opiate Research* (Cambridge, MA: Harvard University Press, 1989), 6–10, 18–21, 24–27, 47–49, 52–63, 188–191.

Robert Kanigel, *Apprentice to Genius: The Making of a Scientific Dynasty* (Baltimore: Johns Hopkins University Press, 1986), x, xiii–xiv, 7–8, 56, 59–63, 122–125, 130–131, 141–142, 157–164, 166–182, 230–233.

Chapter Two: *Shaina Maidel*

Author's interviews with Nancy Marriott, December 16, 2016; January 27–28, 2017; March 11, 2022; April 8, 2022.

Author's interviews with Agu Pert, July 9, 2019; March 18, 2022; July 1, 2022; July 9, 2022.

Author's interviews with Deane Beebe Fitzgerald, September 24, 2019; April 2, 2022; April 9, 2022.

Author's interviews with Nancy Glasser Morris, April 11, 2022; July 22, 2022; August 13, 2022; November 21, 2022.

Author's interview with David and Penny Glasser, April 29, 2022.

Author's interview with Steve Bitel, April 2, 2022.

Candace Pert, "CBP May 2005 Confidential Biosketch," May 2005.

Agu Pert, "Candy," a history of their relationship written for his children, July 2022.

Candace Pert, *Molecules of Emotion: Why You Feel the Way You Feel* (New York: Scribner, 1997), 35–37.

Candace Pert, *Everything You Need to Know to Feel Go(o)d* (Carlsbad, CA: Hay House, 2006), 102–103, 142.

Robert Kanigel, *Apprentice to Genius: The Making of a Scientific Dynasty* (Baltimore: Johns Hopkins University Press, 1986), 166.

Chapter Three: The Prince

Author's interview with Adele Snowman, September 3, 2021.

Author's interviews with Agu Pert, July 9, 2019; March 18, 2022; July 1, 2022; July 9, 2022.

Author's interviews with Edythe London, December 23, 2019; August 31, 2021; October 10, 2022.

Author's interview with Miles Herkenham, July 10, 2019.

Candace Pert, *Molecules of Emotion: Why You Feel the Way You Feel* (New York: Scribner, 1997), 61–62, 73–76, 79–80, 86–89, 92–93, 100–102, 106–117.

Solomon H. Snyder, *Brainstorming: The Science and Politics of Opiate Research* (Cambridge, MA: Harvard University Press, 1989), 63, 67–75, 83–85, 92–94, 97–100, 102–119, 128, 130, 132–133, 136–137, 140–143.

Robert Kanigel, *Apprentice to Genius: The Making of a Scientific Dynasty* (Baltimore: Johns Hopkins University Press, 1986), 182–189, 193–203, 208–211, 215–218, 224, 226.

Candace B. Pert and Solomon H. Snyder, "Opiate Receptor: Demonstration in Nervous Tissue," *Science* 179, no. 4077 (March 9, 1973): 1011–1014.

Beryl Lieff Benderly, "A Complex Social Process," *Science*, September 23, 2013.

Eugene Garfield, "Current Comments: "Controversies Over Opiate Receptor Research Typify Problems Facing Awards Committees," *Essays of an Information Scientist* 4, no. 20 (May 14, 1979): 5–18.

William Pollin, "Pert and the Lasker Award," *Science* 204, no. 4388 (April 6, 1979): 8.

Chapter Four: Poison Pill

Author's interview with Betsy Parker, April 5, 2022.

Author's interview with Miles Herkenham, July 10, 2019.

Author's interviews with Nancy Glasser Morris, April 11, 2022; July 22, 2022; August 13, 2022; November 21, 2022.

Author's interviews with Agu Pert, July 9, 2019; March 18, 2022; July 1, 2022; July 9, 2022.

Author's interview with David and Penny Glasser, April 29, 2022.

Author's interviews with Deane Beebe Fitzgerald, September 24, 2019; April 2, 2022; April 9, 2022.

Author's interviews with Deborah Stokes, May 29, 2019; August 22, 2021.

Author's interview with Anne Young, September 23, 2019.

Candace Pert, *Molecules of Emotion: Why You Feel the Way You Feel* (New York: Scribner, 1997), 118–125, 148–157.

Author's interview with Michael Ruff, January 27, 2017.

Author's interviews with Edythe London, December 23, 2019; August 31, 2021; October 10, 2022.

Robert Kanigel, *Apprentice to Genius: The Making of a Scientific Dynasty* (Baltimore: Johns Hopkins University Press, 1986), 205–206.

Matthew B. Ross, Britta M. Glennon, Raviv Murciano-Goroff, Enrico G. Berkes, Bruce A. Weinberg, and Julia I. Lane, "Women Are Credited Less in Science than Men," *Nature* 608, no. 7921 (June 22, 2022): 135–145.

Garrett Epps, "Brains and Ambition," *Washington Post Magazine*, November 11, 1979.

Chapter Five: "The Crazies"

Author's interviews with Nancy Marriott, December 16, 2016; January 27–28, 2017; March 11, 2022; April 8, 2022.

Author's interviews with Deane Beebe Fitzgerald, September 24, 2019; April 2, 2022; April 9, 2022.

Author's interview with Anne Young, September 23, 2019.

Author's interviews with Edythe London, December 23, 2019; August 31, 2021; October 10, 2022.

Author's interviews with Michael Ruff, December 30, 2016; January 27–28, 2017; March 2, 2017; February 24, 2019; July 5, 2019; July 30, 2019; September 30, 2019; November 11, 2019; November 22, 2019; December 16, 2020; January 17, 2021; August 24, 2021; March 8, 2022.

Author's interviews with Lydia Temoshok, August 7, 2019; August 23, 2019; October 22, 2019; June 19, 2020; December 30, 2020; December 28, 2021; June 27, 2022.

Author's interview with Miles Herkenham, July 10, 2019.

Author's interviews with Agu Pert, July 9, 2019; March 18, 2022; July 1, 2022; July 9, 2022.

Author's interview with Steve Paul, May 20, 2022.

Author's interview with Betsy Parker, April 5, 2022.

Candace Pert, *Molecules of Emotion: Why You Feel the Way You Feel* (New York: Scribner, 1997), 155–158, 165–166.

Kay Redfield Jamison, *Touched with Fire: Manic-Depressive Illness and the Artistic Temperament* (New York: Simon & Schuster, 1993), 103, 105.

Garrett Epps, "Brains and Ambition," *Washington Post Magazine*, November 11, 1979.

Garrett Epps, "Brainstormer: Dr. Candace Pert," *Washington Post*, December 31, 1978.

Chapter Six: Bodymind

Author's interviews with Agu Pert, July 9, 2019; March 18, 2022; July 1, 2022; July 9, 2022.

Author's interviews with Nancy Glasser Morris, April 11, 2022; July 22, 2022; August 13, 2022; November 21, 2022.

Author's interviews with Deane Beebe Fitzgerald, September 24, 2019; April 2, 2022; April 9, 2022.

Author's interviews with Michael Ruff, December 30, 2016; January 27–28, 2017; March 2, 2017; February 24, 2019; July 5, 2019; July 30, 2019; September 30, 2019; November 11, 2019; November 22, 2019; December 16, 2020; January 17, 2021; August 24, 2021; March 8, 2022.

Candace Pert, *Molecules of Emotion: Why You Feel the Way You Feel* (New York: Scribner, 1997), 18, 139–143, 147–148, 159–165, 172–173, 176–178, 181–190, 215, 245, 267–277, 304, 306–307.

Candace Pert, *Everything You Need to Know to Feel Go(o)d* (Carlsbad, CA: Hay House, 2006), 32–36, 43–48, 54, 61–62, 80, 169–171.

Robert Kanigel, *Apprentice to Genius: The Making of a Scientific Dynasty* (Baltimore: Johns Hopkins University Press, 1986), 45.

Justin Skirry, "René Descartes: The Mind-Body Distinction," *Internet Encyclopedia of Philosophy*, https://iep.utm.edu/rene-descartes-mind-body-distinction-dualism (accessed April 23, 2023).

Santiago Moratto, "Theism and Science Inextricably Conjoined," St. Francis & the Americas, Hispanic Research Center, Arizona State University, November 18, 2016, https://stfrancis.clas.asu.edu/article/theism-and-science-inextricably-conjoined.

Emily Eakin, "I Feel, Therefore I Am," *New York Times*, April 19, 2003.

Sally Squires, "Molecules of Emotion," *Washington Post*, August 21, 1985.

Stephen S. Hall, "A Molecular Code Links Emotions, Mind and Health," *Smithsonian*, June 1989.

Chapter Seven: The Plague

Author's interviews with Michael Ruff, December 30, 2016; January 27–28, 2017; March 2, 2017; February 24, 2019; July 5, 2019; July 30, 2019; September 30, 2019; November 11, 2019; November 22, 2019; December 16, 2020; January 17, 2021; August 24, 2021; March 8, 2022.

Author's interviews with Frank Ruscetti, August 8, 2019; May 3, 2022; June 30, 2022.

Author's interviews with Lydia Temoshok, August 7, 2019; August 23, 2019; October 22, 2019; June 19, 2020; December 30, 2020; December 28, 2021; June 27, 2022.

Author's interview with Miles Herkenham, July 10, 2019.

Candace Pert, *Molecules of Emotion: Why You Feel the Way You Feel* (New York: Scribner, 1997), 196–200, 202–207, 215.

Candace Pert, *Everything You Need to Know to Feel Go(o)d* (Carlsbad, CA: Hay House, 2006), 14–16, 213, 215–216.

Candace Pert, letter to Dr. Frank Lilly, President's Commission on the HIV Epidemic, December 16, 1987.

Randy Shilts, *And the Band Played On: Politics, People, and the AIDS Epidemic* (New York: St. Martin's Griffin, 1987), 43–44, 55, 71, 93–95, 110, 143–145, 173–174, 186–187, 191, 207, 214, 224, 235–236, 249, 299–301, 322, 347, 478–479, 513, 554.

Peter Staley, *Never Silent: ACT UP and My Life in Activism* (Chicago: Chicago Review Press, 2022), 66, 75, 82, 117–118.

Garrett Epps, "Brains and Ambition," *Washington Post Magazine*, November 11, 1979.

Harold M. Schmeck Jr., "Research Suggests New AIDS Weapon," *New York Times*, December 16, 1986.

Sally Squires, "AIDS-Blocking Protein Identified," *Washington Post*, December 10, 1986.

Gina Kolata, "Clinical Trials Planned for New AIDS Drug," *Science* 235, no. 4793 (March 6, 1987): 1138–1139.

Jean L. Marx, "Probing the AIDS Virus and Its Relatives," *Science* 236, no. 4808 (June 19, 1987): 1523–1525.

"AIDS: Anatomy of a Discovery, an Interview with Candace Pert," *Science Impact*, June 1987.

Peter Newmark, "AIDS Drug Trials to Start amid Controversy," *Nature* 327, no. 6122 (June 11, 1987): 449.

Alun Anderson, "AIDS Workers Back on Speaking Terms," *Nature* 328, no. 6126 (July 9–15, 1987): 102.

"The Drug Development Process," FDA, January 4, 2018, https://www.fda.gov/patients/learn-about-drug-and-device-approvals/drug-development-process.

"How Drugs Are Developed and Approved," FDA, October 24, 2022, https://www.fda.gov/drugs/development-approval-process-drugs/how-drugs-are-developed-and-approved.

L. Wetterberg, B. Alexius, J. Sääf, A. Sönnerborg, S. Britton, and C. Pert, "Peptide T in Treatment of AIDS," *The Lancet* 329, no. 8525 (January 17, 1987): 159.

J. A. Marcusson, D. Lazega, C. Pert, M. Ruff, K. G. Sundquist, and L. Wetterberg, "Peptide T and Psoriasis," *Acta Dermato-Venereologica Supplementum* (Stockholm) 146 (1989): 117–121.

J. A. Marcusson and L. Wetterberg, "Peptide T in the Treatment of Psoriasis and Psoriatic Arthritis. A Case Report," *Acta Dermato-Venereologica Supplementum* (Stockholm) 69, no. 1 (1989): 86–88.

"Biological, Clinical Improvements Noted in Some Subjects, Peptide T Not Toxic in Phase I Trials," *CDC AIDS Weekly*, June 20, 1988.

Mark Harrington, Jim Eigo, David Z. Kirschenbaum, and Iris Long, "A Glossary of AIDS Drug Trials, Testing & Treatment Issues," ACT UP New York, July 5, 1988.

Celia Hooper, "Potential AIDS Drug Passes First Tests," *Science Today*, July 27, 1988.

Joanna M. Hill, "Peptide T Studied as Anti-AIDS Drug," *Psychiatric Times* 5, no. 7 (July 1998).

Chapter Eight: Failure to Replicate

Author's interviews with Michael Ruff, December 30, 2016; January 27–28, 2017; March 2, 2017; February 24, 2019; July 5, 2019; July 30, 2019;

September 30, 2019; November 11, 2019; November 22, 2019; December 16, 2020; January 17, 2021; August 24, 2021; March 8, 2022.

Author's interviews with Frank Ruscetti, August 8, 2019; May 3, 2022; June 30, 2022.

Author's interview with Jim Mullins, March 30, 2022.

Candace Pert, *Molecules of Emotion: Why You Feel the Way You Feel* (New York: Scribner, 1997), 19, 217–218, 223.

Candace Pert, *Everything You Need to Know to Feel Go(o)d* (Carlsbad, CA: Hay House, 2006), 17.

Candace Pert, letter to Dr. Frank Lilly, President's Commission on the HIV Epidemic, December 16, 1987.

Randy Shilts, *And the Band Played On: Politics, People, and the AIDS Epidemic* (New York: St. Martin's Griffin, 1987), 73–74, 151, 162, 193, 201–202, 219–221, 229, 237, 240, 263–264, 269–271, 289, 319, 334, 349, 366–368, 371–372, 386–388, 409, 419–420, 429–430, 434–435, 448, 451–452, 460–461, 495–497, 528–530, 578, 587–589, 592–594, 597.

Lawrence K. Altman, "French Sue U.S. over AIDS Virus Discovery," *New York Times*, December 14, 1985.

Harold M. Schmeck Jr., "Research Suggests New AIDS Weapon," *New York Times*, December 16, 1986.

Sally Squires, "AIDS-Blocking Protein Identified," *Washington Post*, December 10, 1986.

"Scientists Uncertain About New Drug," *New Scientist*, May 28, 1987.

Jean L. Marx, "Probing the AIDS Virus and Its Relatives," *Science* 236, no. 4808 (June 19, 1987): 1523–1525.

D. M. Barnes, "Debate over Potential AIDS Drug," *Science* 237, no. 4811 (July 10, 1987): 128–130.

Larry Thompson, "Another Drug Controversy Surfaces," *Washington Post*, June 5, 1987.

Peter Newmark, "AIDS Drug Trials to Start amid Controversy," *Nature* 327, no. 6122 (June 11, 1987): 449.

Ron Dagani, "Controversy Surrounds New AIDS Drug Called Peptide T," *Chemical & Engineering News*, July 20, 1987.

"New Trial of Peptide T Begins," *New Scientist* 116, no. 1586 (November 12, 1987): 26.

Marlene Cimons, "AIDS Drug Will Be Tested on Humans," *Philadelphia Inquirer*, November 19, 1987.

Jamie Talan, "Trials in Calif. on AIDS Drug," *Newsday*, November 27, 1987.

"University of Southern California Peptide-T Tests Begin," *CDC AIDS Weekly*, December 21, 1987.

Larry Thompson and Sally Squires, "Treatments and Vaccines: A Status Report," *Washington Post*, January 19, 1988.

Sally Squires, "Scientists Seek to Explain AIDS Dementia," *Washington Post*, February 16, 1988.

Philip M. Boffey, "From Infection to Illness: A Virus's Advancing Toll," *New York Times*, February 14, 1988.

Barry Werth, "The AIDS Windfall," *New England Monthly*, June 1988.

Cecelia Hooper, "The Assault on AIDS," *Detroit News*, August 18, 1988.

"Peptide T Shows Promise as Anti-AIDS Drug," *Los Angeles Times*, August 14, 1988.

R. Weiss, "HIV: More Tricks Up Its Sleeve," *Science News* 134, no. 16 (October 15, 1988): 244.

Steve Rose, "Peptide T: Another Promising AIDS Treatment Enters the Bureaucracy," *Next*, December 7, 1988.

"Peptide T Phase I Trial Shows 'Total Absence' of Toxicity in 12 AIDS Patients, NIMH Scientist Reports," *The Blue Sheet: Health Policy and Biomedical Research News of the Week*, January 18, 1989.

"Peptide T Research Is Impeded Because Researchers Cannot Obtain GP120 Reagent—Investigator Contends," *The Blue Sheet: Health Policy and Biomedical Research News of the Week*, January 18, 1989.

Susan Okie, "Tests of New AIDS Drug Encourage Researchers," *Washington Post*, January 19, 1989.

"New AIDS Drugs on the Horizon," *Insight*, March 6, 1989.

Richard A. Knox, "Anti-AIDS Drug to Be Tested on Fenway Clients," *Boston Globe*, March 29, 1989.

David Smyth, "New Drug Research to Be Expanded: Peptide-T Called 'Promising,'" *Bay Area Reporter*, April 6, 1989.

Masha Gessen, "Rooting for the Underdog," *Next*, September 6, 1989.

David Smyth, "Bristol-Myers Backs Out of Peptide T," *Bay Area Reporter*, July 20, 1989.

"Bristol-Myers Promises Wider Distribution of ddI," *Next*, July 19, 1989.

Peter Erbland, "How Effective Is Peptide T?," *Bay Windows*, July 20–26, 1989.

"Peptide T Phase I Study: Neuropsychiatric Results," *CDC AIDS Weekly*, August 14, 1989.

Seth Rolbein, "Peptide T and the AIDS Establishment," *Boston Magazine*, June 1990.

John Crewdson, "Gallo Admits French Discovered AIDS Virus," *Chicago Tribune*, May 30, 1991.

John Crewdson, "U.S.: Top AIDS Scientist Guilty of Misconduct," *Chicago Tribune*, December 31, 1992.

Jonathan Bor and Douglas Birch, "Scientist Battle State Funding for Gallo Misconduct Charges Reiterated; Researcher Calls Critics 'Fanatics,'" *Baltimore Sun*, November 4, 1995.

Andy Coghlan, "Was Robert Gallo Robbed of the Nobel Prize?," *New Scientist*, October 7, 2008.

Alice Park, "The Story Behind the First AIDS Drug," *Time*, March 19, 2017.

"How the Discovery of HIV Led to a Transatlantic Research War," *PBS NewsHour*, March 24, 2020.

Chapter Nine: Black Market Candy

Author's interviews with Michael Ruff, December 30, 2016; January 27–28, 2017; March 2, 2017; February 24, 2019; July 5, 2019; July 30, 2019; September 30, 2019; November 11, 2019; November 22, 2019; December 16, 2020; January 17, 2021; August 24, 2021; March 8, 2022.

Author's interviews with Evan Pert and Nancy Kingcaid, September 9, 2019; October 28, 2019; March 3, 2021; April 30, 2021; August 4, 2021; November 12, 2021; March 13, 2022; August 5, 2022.

Author's interviews with Vanessa Pert, August 3, 2019; August 23, 2019; September 6, 2019; September 9, 2019; August 26, 2020; January 12, 2021; March 3, 2021; April 30, 2021; August 4, 2021; March 13, 2022; April 2, 2022; August 8, 2022; November 21, 2022.

Author's interviews with Nancy Glasser Morris, April 11, 2022; July 22, 2022; August 13, 2022; November 21, 2022.

Author's interviews with Deane Beebe Fitzgerald, September 24, 2019; April 2, 2022; April 9, 2022.

Author's interview with David and Penny Glasser, April 22, 2022.

Author's interview with Derek Hodel, March 18, 2022.

Author's interview with Garance Franke-Ruta, July 1, 2022.

Garance Franke-Ruta, email to author, July 1, 2022.

Author's interview with Anna Blume, April 22, 2022.

Author's interview with Kenneth Mayer, April 14, 2022.

Candace Pert, *Molecules of Emotion: Why You Feel the Way You Feel* (New York: Scribner, 1997), 231–232.

Candace Pert, *Everything You Need to Know to Feel Go(o)d* (Carlsbad, CA: Hay House, 2006), 127–128.

Randy Shilts, *And the Band Played On: Politics, People, and the AIDS Epidemic* (New York: St. Martin's Griffin, 1987), 563–564.

Peter Staley, *Never Silent: ACT UP and My Life in Activism* (Chicago: Chicago Review Press, 2022), 12–13, 105–106, 115–116, 141, 169.

Gay Men's Health Crisis, "Peptide T," *Treatment Issues: The GMHC Newsletter of Experimental AIDS Therapies* 3, no. 1 (February 6, 1989).

Michael Specter, "New Type of AIDS Drug Holds Promise," *Washington Post*, February 9, 1989.

Andrew Meacham, "New AIDS Drug Shows Promise," *U.S. Journal of Drugs and Alcohol Dependence* 13, no. 3 (March 1989).

Integra Institute and National Institute of Mental Health, "Peptide T Recruitment," excerpt from the Massachusetts Clinical Trials Director for AIDS and HIV-Related Drugs, March 1989.

Richard A. Knox, "Anti-AIDS Drug to Be Tested on Fenway Clients," *Boston Globe*, March 29, 1989.

Susan Brink, "City Clinic to Test New AIDS Drug," *Boston Herald*, March 29, 1989.

Peter Erbland, "Fenway Begins Peptide-T Trials," *Bay Windows*, March 30–April 5, 1989.

National Lesbian and Gay Health Foundation, "Second Peptide T Trial to Begin in Boston," April 5–9, 1989.

"Boston Health Center Will Test Peptide T," *CDC AIDS Weekly*, April 10, 1989.

"Recruitment Begins for Peptide T Study," *Positive Direction News* 2, no. 1 (April–May 1989).

ACT UP New York Treatment + Data Committee, "A Catalogue of AIDS Drug Development Disasters," *Interim Report to the National Committee to Review Current Procedures for Approval of New Drugs for Cancer and AIDS*, May 2, 1989.

"Peptide T and Peptide T (4–8)," *CDC AIDS Weekly*, May 6, 1989.

American Foundation for AIDS Research (amfAR), *AIDS/HIV Experimental Treatment Directory*, May 1989.

ACT UP New York Treatment + Data Committee, ACT UP Boston, ACT UP Provincetown, and Provincetown Positive PWA Coalition, letter to Dr. Anthony Fauci, October 5, 1989.

Cynthia Crossen, "Shock Troops: AIDS Activist Group Harasses and Provokes to Make Its Point," *Wall Street Journal*, December 8, 1989.

Carole Moussalli, "Peptide T: Drug Blocks HIV Attachment to CD4 Receptors," AIDS Patient Care, October 1989.

Candace Pert, letter to Anthony Fauci, December 5, 1989.

Peptide T Study Staff, Fenway Community Health Center, "Don't Dismiss Peptide T," letter to the editor, Bay Windows, February 1, 1990.

Arthur S. Levine, Scientific Director, National Institute of Child Health and Human Development, Department of Health and Human Services, "Status of Investigations on VIP, Peptide T and GP-120 (HIV)," letter to Philip G. Nelson, Chief, Laboratory of Developmental Neurobiology, March 16, 1990.

"AIDS Activists Win Peptide T Treatment," Journal of NIH Research, June 1990.

Anna Blume, "A Chronological History of Peptide T," January 7, 1991.

Gay Men's Health Crisis, "Peptide T Access Blocked," Treatment Issues: The GMHC Newsletter of Experimental AIDS Therapies 5, no. 1 (January 10, 1991).

Chapter Ten: Squeaky Clean

Author's interviews with Michael Ruff, December 30, 2016; January 27–28, 2017; March 2, 2017; February 24, 2019; July 5, 2019; July 30, 2019; September 30, 2019; November 11, 2019; November 22, 2019; December 16, 2020; January 17, 2021; August 24, 2021; March 8, 2022.

Author's interviews with Jeffrey Galpin, November 14, 2019; January 16, 2021; July 21, 2022; August 5, 2022.

Author's interviews with Peter Heseltine, October 22, 2019; March 18, 2022.

Author's interview with Peter Bridge, April 21, 2022.

Peter Heseltine, email to author, April 11, 2022.

J. Hampton Atkinson, email to author, April 13, 2022.

Robert K. Heaton, emails to author, April 6, 2022; April 10, 2022.

Karl Goodkin, email to author, May 24, 2022.

Candace Pert, Molecules of Emotion: Why You Feel the Way You Feel (New York: Scribner, 1997), 219, 226–228, 230–231, 247–249.

Candace Pert, Everything You Need to Know to Feel Go(o)d (Carlsbad, CA: Hay House, 2006), 126–127, 129–131.

Sally Squires, "Scientists Seek to Explain AIDS Dementia," Washington Post, February 16, 1989.

"Bristol-Myers to Get Rights to Market New AIDS Drug," Wall Street Journal, March 2, 1988.

Reuters, "U.S. to Let Bristol-Myers Market AIDS Drug," *New York Times*, March 13, 1988.

Gina Kolata, "The Evolving Biology of AIDS: Scavenger Cell Looms Large," *New York Times*, June 7, 1988.

Marilyn Chase, "Scientists Present Data on Possible AIDS Treatments," *Wall Street Journal*, June 16, 1988.

David Smyth, "Bristol-Myers Signs License for AIDS Drug," *San Francisco Sentinel*, August 26, 1988.

Harold M. Schmeck Jr., "Studies Link AIDS Virus Directly to Cancer and Dementia," *New York Times*, October 18, 1988.

"Pert and Partner Take Peptide Proves Private," *NIMH Record*, November 15, 1988.

Office of Communications, National Institute of Allergy and Infectious Diseases, "Joint NIMH-NIAID Statement on Peptide T," AIDS Clinical Trials Alert, December 18, 1989.

"NIMH, NIAID Suggest Controlled Double Blind Peptide T Study," *NIAID AIDS Agenda*, January 1990.

Anthony Fauci, letter to Candace Pert, January 2, 1990.

Candace Pert, letter to Anthony Fauci, March 29, 1990.

Candace Pert, "Commentary: A Crime Far Worse than Fraud Threatens Scientific Progress," *The Scientist*, April 2, 1990.

Candace Pert, "Peptide T in Phase II," *PWA Coalition Newsline*, no. 77, June 1992.

Neenyah Ostrom, "Peptide T Enters Phase II Testing," *New York Native*, no. 508, January 11, 1993.

National Institutes of Health, National Institute of Mental Health, "Analyses of Peptide T Efficacy on Neuropsychological Performance in HIV Seropositive Individuals with Cognitive Impairment," NIMH press release, October 24, 1995.

Peter N. R. Heseltine, Karl Goodkin, J. Hampton Atkinson, Benedetto Vitiello, James Rochon, Robert K. Heaton, Ealaine M. Eaton, Frances L. Wilkie, Eugene Sobel, Stephen J. Brown, Dan Feaster, Lon Schneider, Walter L. Goldschmidts, and Ellen S. Stover, "Randomized Double-Blind Placebo-Controlled Trial of Peptide T for HIV-Associated Cognitive Impairment," *Archives of Neurology* 55, no. 1 (January 1998): 41–51.

George Grimes, "Notes from NIH Pharmacy Indicating Gelling of Study Medication 'Peptide T' (DAPTA)," March 25, 1991; November 17, 1994, revision.

Luke Adams, "The Other Secret of NIMH: Feds Misled Public on Peptide T," *Bay Area Reporter*, October 9, 1998.

Chapter Eleven: Spirit of Truth

Author's interviews with Michael Ruff, December 30, 2016; January 27–28, 2017; March 2, 2017; February 24, 2019; July 5, 2019; July 30, 2019; September 30, 2019; November 11, 2019; November 22, 2019; December 16, 2020; January 17, 2021; August 24, 2021; March 8, 2022.

Author's interviews with Peter Heseltine, October 22, 2019; March 18, 2022.

Author's interview with Steve Paul, May 20, 2022.

Candace Pert, *Molecules of Emotion: Why You Feel the Way You Feel* (New York: Scribner, 1997), 186–188, 221–222, 234–235, 237–238, 240–246, 274–276, 296, 304, 310–315.

Candace Pert, *Everything You Need to Know to Feel Go(o)d* (Carlsbad, CA: Hay House, 2006), 57, 98–101, 114, 119, 147, 151–152, 156–157, 162–164, 182–183, 192–193, 215.

Robert Kanigel, *Apprentice to Genius: The Making of a Scientific Dynasty* (Baltimore: Johns Hopkins University Press, 1986), 248, 252.

Karl Goodkin, Benedetto Vitiello, William D. Lyman, Deshatn Asthana, J. Hampton Atkinson, Peter N. R. Heseltine, Rebeca Molina, Wenli Zheng, Imad Khamis, Frances L. Wilkie, and Paul Shapshak, "Cerebrospinal and Peripheral Human Immunodeficiency Virus Type 1 Load in a Multisite, Randomized, Double-Blind, Placebo-Controlled Trial of D-Ala1-Peptide T-Amide for HIV-1-Associated Cognitive-Motor Impairment," *Journal of NeuroVirology* 12, no. 3 (June 2006): 178–189.

Candace Pert, letter to Eckart Wintzen, August 2002.

Candace Pert, statement on AIDS Treatment Activists Coalition (ATAC) listserv, January 2003.

Mark Harrington, statements on AIDS Treatment Activists Coalition (ATAC) listserv, January 2003.

Dylan Matthews, "What 'Dallas Buyers Club' Got Wrong About the AIDS Crisis," *Washington Post*, December 10, 2013.

Peter Staley, *Never Silent: ACT UP and My Life in Activism* (Chicago: Chicago Review Press, 2022), 226, 228–229.

Solomon H. Snyder, *Brainstorming: The Science and Politics of Opiate Research* (Cambridge, MA: Harvard University Press, 1989), 140–143.

"Overdose Death Rates," National Institute on Drug Abuse, February 9, 2023, https://nida.nih.gov/research-topics/trends-statistics/overdose-death-rates.

"The Drug Overdose Epidemic: Behind the Numbers," Centers for Disease Control and Prevention, https://www.cdc.gov/opioids/data/index.html (last reviewed June 1, 2020).

Kevin E. Vowles, Mindy L. McEntee, Peter Siyahhan Julnes, Tessa Frohe, John P. Ney, and David N. van der Goes, "Rates of Opioid Misuse, Abuse, and Addiction in Chronic Pain: A Systematic Review and Data Synthesis," *Pain* 156, no. 4 (April 2015): 569–576.

Curtis S. Florence, Feijun Luo, Likang Xu, and Chao Zhou, "The Economic Burden of Prescription Opioid Overdose Abuse and Dependence in the United States, 2013," *Medical Care* 54, no. 10 (October 2016): 901–906.

John Abramson, *Sickening: How Big Pharma Broke American Health Care and How We Can Repair It* (Boston: Mariner Books, 2022), 110–113, 123–124, 154–157.

Albert Rothenberg, "Creative Cognitive Processes in Kekulé's Discovery of the Structure of the Benzene Molecule," *American Journal of Psychology* 108, no. 3 (Autumn 1995): 419–438.

"August Kekulé," *Wikipedia*, https://en.wikipedia.org/wiki/August_Kekulé (page last edited March 14, 2023).

Alli N. McCoy and Siang Yong Tan, "Otto Loewi (1873–1961): Dreamer and Nobel Laureate," *Singapore Medical Journal* 55, no 1 (January 2014): 3–4.

Michelle Feder, "Dmitri Mendeleev, Building the Periodic Table of Elements," Khan Academy, https://www.khanacademy.org/humanities/big-history-project/stars-and-elements/knowing-stars-elements/a/dmitri-mendeleev.

Maria Popova, "How Dmitri Mendeleev His Periodic Table in a Dream," *The Marginalian*, February 8, 2016, https://www.themarginalian.org/2016/02/08/mendeleev-periodic-table-dream/.

Anthony Gottlieb, "What Did Descartes Really Know?," *New Yorker*, November 20, 2006.

Justin Skirry, "René Descartes: The Mind-Body Distinction," *Internet Encyclopedia of Philosophy*, https://iep.utm.edu/rene-descartes-mind-body-distinction-dualism (accessed April 23, 2023).

Santiago Moratto, "Theism and Science Inextricably Conjoined," St. Francis & the Americas, Hispanic Research Center, Arizona State University, November 18, 2016, https://stfrancis.clas.asu.edu/article/theism-and-science-inextricably-conjoined.

Candace Pert, "Molecules of Emotion: Emotions as Information Resolving Mind-Body Duality," lecture presented at Tendrel "Unity in Duality" Conference, Munich, October 2002.

Bonnie Horrigan, "Candace Pert, PhD: Neuropeptides, AIDS and the Science of Mind-Body Healing," *Alternative Therapies in Health and Medicine* 1, no. 3 (July 1995): 70–76.

Chapter Twelve: The C-Word

Author's interview with Steve Paul, May 20, 2022.

Author's interviews with Michael Ruff, December 30, 2016; January 27–28, 2017; March 2, 2017; February 24, 2019; July 5, 2019; July 30, 2019; September 30, 2019; November 11, 2019; November 22, 2019; December 16, 2020; January 17, 2021; August 24, 2021; March 8, 2022.

Author's interviews with Edythe London, December 23, 2019; August 31, 2021; October 10, 2022.

Author's interviews with Vivian Komori, October 3, 2019; October 8, 2019; November 12, 2019; August 26, 2020; March 19, 2022; April 5, 2022; April 14, 2022.

Author's interviews with Mark Lloyd-Fox, October 21, 2019; January 3, 2021.

Author's interviews with Jeffrey Galpin, November 14, 2019; January 16, 2021; July 21, 2022; August 5, 2022.

Author's interview with Austin Vickers, September 9, 2019.

Agreement Between Rapid Pharmaceuticals AG, Vivian Komori, Gardner Holding AG, Candace B. Pert, and Michael R. Ruff, September 5, 2007.

Shareholder Agreement Between Gardner Holding AG, Zug, Candace B. Pert, Michael R. Ruff, and Vivian Komori, January 5, 2008.

Addendum to Shareholder Agreement Between Gardner Holding AG, Zug, Candace B. Pert, Michael R. Ruff, and Vivian Komori, July 1, 2008.

Addendum to Shareholder Agreement Between Gardner Holding AG, Zug, Candace B. Pert, Michael R. Ruff, and Vivian Komori, October 18, 2010.

Agreement and Plan of Reorganization Between Gardner Holding AG, Zug, Candace B. Pert, Michael R. Ruff, and Vivian Komori, January 5, 2008.

Candace Pert, Confidentiality and Invention Assignment Agreement, May 1, 2008.

Michael Ruff, Confidentiality and Invention Assignment Agreement, May 1, 2008.

Mark Lloyd-Fox, email to Michael Laznicka, June 9, 2008.

Mark Lloyd-Fox, email and proposal to Michael Laznicka re: Rapid Pharmaceuticals Director of Government Relations and Public Affairs, September 3, 2008.

Michael Laznicka, email to Mark Lloyd-Fox, September 9, 2008.

Michael Laznicka, email to Mark Lloyd-Fox with Certificate Purchase Agreement Between Gardner Holding AG and Mark Lloyd-Fox, September 11, 2008.

Mark Lloyd-Fox, Draft Proposal for Contractual Agreements Between Michael Laznicka and Jason Andrew Mark Lloyd-Fox re: Rapid Pharmaceuticals Director of Government Affairs and Public Relations position, September 15, 2008.

Michael Laznicka, Finder's Agreement Between Gardner Holding AG and Mark Lloyd-Fox, January 1, 2009.

Prof. Dr. Jur. Georg Jochum, Apl. Prof. An Der University Konstanz, Rechtsanwalt, Rapid Pharmaceuticals AZ, Zug, Enterprise Value Assessment Certification, January 5, 2009.

Christoph Jochum MD, University of Duisberg-Essen, Scientific Expert's Assessment on Monomeric DAPTA, January 19, 2009.

Michael Laznicka, CEO, Rapid Pharmaceuticals, Internal Business Plan, Zug, Versions 0.7 and 0.8, February 2009.

Rapid Pharmaceuticals, HIV/AIDS and Psoriasis Therapy, Business Overview, June 2009.

Rapid Pharmaceuticals, Company Business Plan, Version 1.2, June 2009.

Rapid Pharmaceuticals Executive Summary, June 2009.

Michael Laznicka, Finder's Agreement Between Rapid Pharmaceuticals AG and Mark Lloyd-Fox, June 2009.

Rapid Master Agreement of Summer 2012 Between Candace Pert, Michael Ruff, and Gardner Holding AG, August 15, 2012.

Defendants' Answer, Affirmative Defenses, and Counterclaims, *Rapid Pharmaceuticals AG v. Kachroo et al.,* United States District Court, District of Massachusetts, 1:15-cv-13161-NMG, October 13, 2015.

Minutes of the Board of Directors Meeting of Rapid Pharmaceuticals AG, March 23, 2015.

Gaytri Kachroo, letter to Lisa A. Haile, Partner, DLA Piper LLP (US), March 2017.

Vivian Komori, email to Lisa A. Haile and Thiru Vignarajah, Partners, DLA Piper LLP (US), March 21, 2017.

Chapter Thirteen: The Travesty Tour

Author's interviews with Michael Ruff, December 30, 2016; January 27–28, 2017; March 2, 2017; February 24, 2019; July 5, 2019; July 30, 2019; September 30, 2019; November 11, 2019; November 22, 2019; December 16, 2020; January 17, 2021; August 24, 2021; March 8, 2022.

Author's interviews with Mark Lloyd-Fox, October 21, 2019; January 3, 2021.

Author's interviews with Nancy Glasser Morris, April 11, 2022; July 22, 2022; August 13, 2022; November 21, 2022.

Author's interviews with Jane Barrash, May 29, 2019; August 9, 2019.

Author's interviews with Deborah Stokes, May 29, 2019; August 9, 2019; August 22, 2021.

Author's interviews with Lydia Temoshok, August 7, 2019; August 23, 2019; October 22, 2019; June 19, 2020; December 30, 2020; December 28, 2021; June 27, 2022.

Author's interviews with Vanessa Pert, August 3, 2019; August 23, 2019; September 6, 2019; September 9, 2019; August 26, 2020; January 12, 2021; March 3, 2021; April 30, 2021; August 4, 2021; March 13, 2022; April 2, 2022; August 8, 2022; November 21, 2022.

Candace Pert, "CBP May 2005 Confidential Biosketch," May 2005.

Author's interviews with Evan Pert and Nancy Kingcaid, September 9, 2019; October 28, 2019; March 3, 2021; April 30, 2021; August 4, 2021; November 12, 2021; March 13, 2022; August 5, 2022.

Author's interviews with Deane Beebe Fitzgerald, September 24, 2019; April 2, 2022; April 9, 2022.

Author's interviews with Nancy Marriott, December 16, 2016; January 27–28, 2017; March 11, 2022; April 8, 2022.

Michael Ruff, "Love Remembrance," Wynne Ilene Beebe Service of Thanksgiving, October 4, 1998.

Candace Pert, *Everything You Need to Know to Feel Go(o)d* (Carlsbad, CA: Hay House, 2006), 131, 138–141, 144.

Chapter Fourteen: Fighting Vipers

Author's interviews with Nancy Glasser Morris, April 11, 2022; July 22, 2022; August 13, 2022; November 21, 2022.

Author's interviews with Michael Ruff, December 30, 2016; January 27–28, 2017; March 2, 2017; February 24, 2019; July 5, 2019; July 30, 2019;

September 30, 2019; November 11, 2019; November 22, 2019; December 16, 2020; January 17, 2021; August 24, 2021; March 8, 2022.

Author's interview with Padma Oza, October 10, 2019.

Author's interviews with Evan Pert and Nancy Kingcaid, September 9, 2019; October 28, 2019; March 3, 2021; April 30, 2021; August 4, 2021; November 12, 2021; March 13, 2022; August 5, 2022.

Author's interviews with Mark Lloyd-Fox, October 21, 2019; January 3, 2021.

Author's interviews with Vivian Komori, October 3, 2019; October 8, 2019; November 12, 2019; August 26, 2020; March 19, 2022; April 5, 2022; April 14, 2022.

Author's interviews with Deborah Stokes, May 29, 2019; August 9, 2019; August 22, 2021.

Bill Ibelle, "The Whistleblower's Lawyer, Gaytri Kachroo S.J.D. '02," *Harvard Law Today*, June 10, 2009.

Candice E. Jackson, attorney for Vivian Komori, email to Michael Laznicka, June 26, 2012.

Gaytri Kachroo, Term Sheet for Master Agreement Between Candace Pert, Michael Ruff, and Gardner Holding AG, August 2012.

Rapid Master Agreement of Summer 2012 Between Candace Pert, Michael Ruff, and Gardner Holding AG, August 15, 2012.

Waiver Regarding 2012 Share Transfer to PC Investors, September 12, 2012.

Gaytri Kachroo, Kachroo Legal Services, PC, Engagement Letter of March 27, 2012.

Gaytri Kachroo on behalf of Venus Ltd. and Lee Kachroo on behalf of Black Squares, Ltd., "Comfort Letter" to Candace Pert and Michael Ruff, July 27, 2012.

Gaytri Kachroo, Full Disclosure and Potential Conflict Waiver Letter to Candace Pert and Michael Ruff, July 28, 2012.

Mutual Release Between Solar Fortune Limited, Gardner Holding AG, Rapid Pharmaceuticals AG, Candace Pert, Michael Ruff, and Vivian Komori, December 7, 2012.

Gaytri Kachroo, Letter to All Rapid Pharmaceuticals AG Shareholders re: Shareholder Letter Number 4, Transition Progress, Operational Items, Funding, and Pharma Partnerships, December 5, 2012.

Operating Agreement of PNR Holdings, LLC, June 14, 2013.

Gaytri Kachroo, Agreement Among Certain Members and Affiliates of PNR Holdings, LLC, June 25, 2013.

Gaytri Kachroo, Chairman and CEO, Rapid Pharmaceuticals, Consulting Agreement with Kirin Kachroo-Levine, Teiresias Consulting, May 6, 2014.

Affidavit of Leeladher Kachroo, November 2, 2015.

Investment Agreement Between Cynthia Ingraham and Rapid Pharmaceuticals AG, August 15, 2013.

Gaytri Kachroo, Agreement Among Certain Members and Affiliates of PNR Holdings, LLC, May 23, 2014.

Candace Pert, email to Michael Ruff, Gaytri Kachroo, Angela Bussio, Mark Lloyd-Fox, and Austin Vickers, September 11, 2013.

Candice E. Jackson, Attorney for Vivian Komori, email to Michael Laznicka and Michael Ruff, July 14, 2015.

Chapter Fifteen: Coming Clean

Author's interviews with Evan Pert and Nancy Kingcaid, September 9, 2019; October 28, 2019; March 3, 2021; April 30, 2021; August 4, 2021; November 12, 2021; March 13, 2022; August 5, 2022.

Author's interviews with Deane Beebe Fitzgerald, September 24, 2019; April 2, 2022; April 9, 2022.

Author's interview with Andrea Schara, October 8, 2019.

Author's interviews with Lydia Temoshok, August 7, 2019; August 23, 2019; October 22, 2019; June 19, 2020; December 30, 2020; December 28, 2021; June 27, 2022.

Author's interviews with Michael Ruff, December 30, 2016; January 27–28, 2017; March 2, 2017; February 24, 2019; July 5, 2019; July 30, 2019; September 30, 2019; November 11, 2019; November 22, 2019; December 16, 2020; January 17, 2021; August 24, 2021; March 8, 2022.

Author's interview with Padma Oza, October 10, 2019.

Author's interviews Mark Lloyd-Fox, October 21, 2019; January 3, 2021.

Author's interviews with Jeffrey Galpin, November 14, 2019; January 16, 2021; July 21, 2022; August 5, 2022.

Author's interviews with Vivian Komori, October 3, 2019; October 8, 2019; November 12, 2019; August 26, 2020; March 19, 2022; April 5, 2022; April 14, 2022.

Candace Pert, *Everything You Need to Know to Feel Go(o)d* (Carlsbad, CA: Hay House, 2006), 228–229.

Bram Zwagemaker, Ex'pert Chairman; Candace Pert, Ex'pert CEO; Michael Ruff, Ex'pert Executive Vice President; Eckart Wintzen, AITI Chairman; MerriBeth Adams, AITI CEO; Dean R. Farrand, AITI Executive Vice President, Ex'pert Agreement, February 19, 2001.

Wayne P. Gulliver, CEO, Advanced Immuni T, email to Candace B. Pert and Michael R. Ruff re: AITI/Georgetown CRADA Termination Notice, December 3, 2004.

Wayne P. Gulliver, CEO, Advanced Immuni T, email and FedEx to Candace B. Pert and Michael R. Ruff re: Consulting Agreement Termination Notice, December 13, 2004.

Feasibility Study Agreement Between Aegis Therapeutics, LLC (Authorized Official: Edward T. Maggio, PhD) and Rapid Pharmaceuticals, Inc. (Authorized Official: Michael Ruff and Rapid's Scientist: Candace Pert), December 22, 2005.

Steven M. Ferguson, Director, Division of Technology Development and Transfer, National Institutes of Health, letter to Wayne P. Gilliver MD, AITI CEO, re: Approval of HIV Peptide T License Assignment, February 23, 2005.

Public Health Service Patent License Agreement—Exclusive, signed by Steven M. Ferguson, Director, Division of Technology Development and Transfer, Office of Technology Transfer, National Institutes of Health, and MerriBeth Adams, February 28, 2006, and March 1, 2006.

Michael Colopy, email to Scott Meza, Candace Pert, and Michael Ruff, subject: Agreement on Proceeding to Settlement, Sublicense Deal Process Points, June 9, 2006.

Peptide T Holdings, Inc. Subject to Contract Re: Proposal for Asset Purchase Transaction between Advanced Peptides & Biotechnology Sciences, Advanced Immuni T, Inc., and Advanced Immuni T Canada, Inc. (Frank Monstrey, Director) and Peptide T Holdings, Inc. (Jeffrey E. Galpin, M.D.), June 9, 2006.

Candace Pert, letter to Mia Prather, Division of Antiviral Drug Products, FDA, May 1, 2008.

Candace Pert, letter to Stacy P. Newalu, PMH, Regulatory Health Project Manager, FDA, May 29, 2009.

Gaytri Kachroo, letter to All Rapid Shareholders & Friends re: Dr. Candace Pert, September 16, 2013.

Minutes of the Board of Directors Meeting of Rapid Pharmaceuticals AG, September 20, 2013.

Assignment of Debt Agreement Between Kachroo Legal Services, P.C., PNR Holdings, LLC, and Rapid Pharmaceuticals AG, September 25, 2013.

Gaytri Kachroo, Management Contract Between Rapid Pharmaceuticals AG and Gaytri Kachroo, May 8, 2014.

Gaytri Kachroo, Board of Directors Contract Between Rapid Pharmaceuticals AG and Gaytri Kachroo, May 8, 2014.

TruthFinder Background Report, Michael Roland Ruff, August 4, 2021.

Contract to Transfer All of the Intellectual Property and Data Owned at Any Time by Peptide T Holdings Ltd. and Brain Matters LLC (Collectively Known as the "Peptide T Companies") to Rapid Pharmaceuticals AG ("Rapid") Effective September 1, 2013, signed by Gaytri Kachroo, Merri-Beth Adams, and Dr. Jeffrey Galpin, December 20, 2013.

Subordinated Loan Agreement Between Kachroo Legal Services, P.C., and Rapid Pharmaceuticals AG, February 17, 2014.

Amendment to Data Transfer Agreement, MerriBeth Adams and Gaytri Kachroo, June 13, 2014.

Gaytri Kachroo, "CEO's Update" to Rapid shareholders, Quarter 4, 2014.

Gaytri Kachroo, Shareholder Letter Number 30, Annual Meeting Notes, December 19, 2014.

Gaytri D. Kachroo, President and Secretary, and Kirin Kachroo-Levine, Treasurer, State of Delaware Annual Franchise Tax Report, 2014.

Gaytri Kachroo, letter to Michael Ruff re: Notice of Termination, February 12, 2015,

Minutes of the Board of Directors Meeting of Rapid Pharmaceuticals AG, March 23, 2015.

Multilateral Settlement Agreement Between Rapid Pharmaceuticals AG, MerriBeth Adams, Peptide T Holdings, Inc., Jeff Galpin, and Certain Investors into Rapid Pharmaceuticals AG (Post-2012 Investors), 2015. Drafted by Gaytri Kachroo and unsigned.

Gaytri Kachroo, "Highly Confidential and Only for PC Investors" letter, April 5, 2015.

Gaytri Kachroo, Business Plan for Arise BioPharma, Inc., April 2015.

Settlement Agreement Between Rapid Pharmaceuticals AG, Pert and Ruff Family Fund, LLC, PnR Holdings, LLC, and the estate of Candace Pert and Michael Ruff, April 15, 2015.

Joint Statement of Michael Ruff and Gaytri Kachroo to the Shareholders of Rapid Pharmaceuticals AG, April 16, 2015.

Share Transfer Between Michael Ruff (PNR Holdings, LLC) and Gaytri Kachroo (Venus Corporation), April 16, 2015.

Michael Ruff, email to Evan Pert and family, April 16, 2015.

Gaytri Kachroo, letter to All Rapid Shareholders re: Restructuring Rapid Pharmaceuticals AG, May 4, 2015.

Gaytri Kachroo, The Reorganization Plan, Draft for Discussion Purposes Only, 2015.

Michael Blume, Partner, and Tobias Wölfle, Senior Manager, KPMG AG Audit, registered/confidential letter to the members of the Board of Directors of Rapid Pharmaceuticals AG, May 21, 2015.

Rapid Pharmaceuticals AG, Capitalization Table Before and After Management Equity, June 3, 2015.

Gaytri Kachroo, Restructuring Plan Version 3, June 8, 2015.

Verified Complaint and Demand for Jury Trial, Circuit Court for Montgomery County, Maryland, *Rapid Pharmaceuticals AG and Rapid Laboratories, Inc. v. Michael Ruff, an individual, and Michael Ruff, Personal Representative of the Estate of Candace Pert and Magic Bullets, LLC*, June 12, 2015.

Lisa A. Haile, Partner, DLA Piper LLP (US), email to Gaytri Kachroo, CEO and Chairman of Rapid Pharmaceuticals AG and Rapid Laboratories, Inc., June 15, 2015.

Gaytri Kachroo, letter to all Rapid shareholders re: Notification of Bankruptcy Filing, June 18, 2015.

Proxy, Michael Ruff Gives Michael Laznicka Right to Fully Represent Him at Extraordinary Shareholders' Meeting on July 3, 2015, June 25, 2015.

Rapid Pharmaceuticals AG, Invitation to the Extraordinary General Meeting of Shareholders, July 3, 2015.

Statement of Vivian Komori—Shareholder of Rapid Pharmaceuticals AG, July 15, 2015.

Statement of Mark Lloyd-Fox—Shareholder of Rapid Pharmaceuticals AG, July 15, 2015.

Statement of Maggieann Miller—Shareholder of Rapid Pharmaceuticals AG, July 15, 2015.

Statement of Evan Pert, Eldest Child of Candace Pert, Shareholder of PNR Holdings LLC and Thereby of Rapid Pharmaceuticals AG, July 15, 2015.

Statement of Jorge Guerra—Senior Clinical Development Advisor and member of the Board of Rapid Pharmaceuticals AG, July 10, 2015.

Cantonal High Court Zug, registered letter to Gaytri Kachroo, August 4, 2015, with decision dated August 13, 2015.

Gaytri Kachroo, memo to Management Team re: Transition and Litigation, September 2, 2015.

Callum Borchers, "Dispute Over HIV Treatment Featured in Movie Sparks Lawsuit," *Boston Globe*, September 16, 2015.

Affidavit of Michael Ruff, *Rapid Pharmaceuticals AG v. Kachroo et al.*, United States District Court, District of Massachusetts, 1:15-cv-13161-NMG, September 18, 2015.

Affidavit of Michael Laznicka, September 23, 2015.

Affidavit of Stephen Kennedy Smith, September 27, 2015.

Affidavit of Gaytri Kachroo, September 28, 2015.

United State District Court, District of Massachusetts, Transcript of Motion Hearing Before the Honorable Marianne B. Bowler, United States Magistrate Judge, *Rapid Pharmaceuticals AG v. Kachroo et al.*, United States District Court, District of Massachusetts, 1:15-cv-13161-NMG, September 30, 2015.

Affidavit of Praveen Tyle, October 2, 2015.

Corey McCann, President of the Board of Directors, Rapid Pharmaceuticals AG, letter re: Declaration of Invalidity to MerriBeth Adams, Jeffrey Galpin, Advanced Immuni T, Inc, Peptide T Holdings, Inc., October 6, 2015.

Affidavit of Roger Hofer in Support of Emergency Motion for Preliminary Injunction, October 8, 2015.

Defendants' Answer, Affirmative Defenses, and Counterclaims, *Rapid Pharmaceuticals AG v. Kachroo et al.*, United States District Court, District of Massachusetts, 1:15-cv-13161-NMG, October 13, 2015.

Affidavit of Robert Fremeau, October 13, 2015.

Affidavit of Detlef Fels, October 13, 2015.

Affidavit of Stephen Kennedy Smith, October 14, 2015.

Affidavit of Gaytri Kachroo, October 28, 2015.

Affidavit of Per Gjorstrup, October 28, 2015.

Affidavit of MerriBeth Adams, October 2015.

Affidavit of Leeladher Kachroo, November 2, 2015.

Affidavit of Suzan Davis, November 2, 2015.

Supplemental Affidavit of Robert Fremeau, November 3, 2015.

Affidavit of Martin Sawitzki, November 4, 2015.

Nathaniel M. Gorton, United States District Judge, United States District Court, District of Massachusetts, Memorandum and Order, December 23, 2015.

Rapid Pharmaceuticals Board of Directors, letter to Shareholders of Rapid Pharmaceuticals AG, February 19, 2016.

United States District Court, District of Massachusetts, Joint Status Report, June 14, 2016.

United States District Court, District of Massachusetts, Defendant Gaytri Kachroo's Statement to the Court, April 17, 2019.

United States District Court, District of Massachusetts, *Rapid Pharmaceuticals AG v. Gaytri Kachroo, et al.*, Before the Honorable Nathaniel M. Gorton, District Judge, April 18, 2019.

Matter of Kachroo, 2020 NY Slip Op 00254, Decided on January 14, 2020, Justia US Law, https://law.justia.com/cases/new-york/appellate-division -first-department/2020/2020-ny-slip-op-00254.html.

"Special Report: Michael Laznicka," *Los Angeles Business Journal*, July 28, 2016.

Board of Bar Overseers, Summary in re: Gaytri D. Kachroo, S.J.C. Judgment Accepting Affidavit of Resignation as a Disciplinary Sanction, entered by Justice Cypher on October 26, 2018.

2020 Annual Report, State of New York First Judicial Department, Attorney Grievance Committee, Supreme Court, Appellate Division, pp. 53–54.

Chapter Sixteen: Release the Spirit

John Abramson, *Sickening: How Big Pharma Broke American Health Care and How We Can Repair It* (Boston: Mariner Books, 2022), 111.

Author's interviews with Michael Ruff, December 30, 2016; January 27–28, 2017; March 2, 2017; February 24, 2019; July 5, 2019; July 30, 2019; September 30, 2019; November 11, 2019; November 22, 2019; December 16, 2020; January 17, 2021; August 24, 2021; March 8, 2022.

Author's interviews with Nancy Glasser Morris, April 11, 2022; July 22, 2022; August 13, 2022; November 21, 2022.

Author's interview with David and Penny Glasser, April 29, 2022.

Author's interviews with Evan Pert and Nancy Kingcaid, September 9, 2019; October 28, 2019; March 3, 2021; April 30, 2021; August 4, 2021; November 12, 2021; March 13, 2022; August 5, 2022.

Author's interviews with Vanessa Pert, August 3, 2019; August 23, 2019; September 6, 2019; September 9, 2019; August 26, 2020; January 12, 2021; March 3, 2021; April 30, 2021; August 4, 2021; March 13, 2022; April 2, 2022; August 8, 2022; November 21, 2022.

Author's interviews with Joe Skinner, July 30, 2019; August 22, 2019.

Author's interview with Zidi Berger, October 28, 2019.

Author's interviews with Deborah Stokes, May 29, 2019; August 9, 2019; August 22, 2021.

Author's interviews with Lydia Temoshok, August 7, 2019; August 23, 2019; October 22, 2019; June 19, 2020; December 30, 2020; December 28, 2021; June 27, 2022.

Author's interview with Austin Vickers, September 19, 2019.

Author's interview with Adam "Omkara" Helfer, August 2, 2021.

Author's interviews with Gilah Rosner, January 27–28, 2017; July 30, 2019.

Author's interview with Andrea Schara, October 8, 2019.

Michael Ruff, email to Deborah Stokes, September 22, 2013; October 17, 2013; November 27, 2013.

Angela Bussio, email to Michael Ruff, Gaytri Kachroo, and Austin Vickers, August 13, 2015.

Gilah Rosner, Facebook post, September 11, 2013; September 16, 2013; December 8, 2016.

Michael Ruff, email to Lydia Temoshok, May 26, 2022.

Epilogue

Author's interviews with Michael Ruff, December 30, 2016; January 27–28, 2017; March 2, 2017; February 24, 2019; July 5, 2019; July 30, 2019; September 30, 2019; November 11, 2019; November 22, 2019; December 16, 2020; January 17, 2021; August 24, 2021; March 8, 2022.

Creative Bio-Peptides, "Preclinical Data Demonstrate Potential of Creative Bio-Peptides' Multi-Chemokine Receptor Antagonist RAP-103 to Enhance Opioid Analgesia and Inhibit Opioid-Derived Dependence, Withdrawal and Respiratory Depression," *Drug and Alcohol Dependence*, September 2022.

Creative Bio-Peptides, "RAP-103 Benefits in Pain Published," *Life Sciences*, July 2022.

ACKNOWLEDGMENTS

THIS BOOK WOULD NOT HAVE BEEN POSSIBLE WITHOUT MY AGENT, EILEEN COPE, whose tireless devotion and encouragement propelled me forward. I am profoundly grateful for her intelligence, loyalty, advocacy, and friendship; she has gone above and beyond in every way.

I feel deep appreciation for the team at Hachette Books, particularly my gifted editor, Lauren Marino, who stuck with me even when the story I'd intended to tell became a different story entirely. Her vision and insight shaped a complex tale. Thank you as well to Mary Ann Naples for taking a risk, to Niyati Patel for keeping us on track, and to Julie Checkoway, whose discerning comments on my proposal made all the difference.

I am also thankful for my legal team, especially my longtime entertainment attorney and friend Nicole Page, as well as Julie Ford, Kay Murray, Rebecca LeGrand, and Greg Lipper, for their counsel and direction. And for Herman Weisberg, a sage sounding board and advisor.

ACKNOWLEDGMENTS

This project began in 2015 when Marilyn Horowitz suggested I read *Molecules of Emotion* as background research for a separate script; little did I know Candace's story would become my main event. It took off after a synchronistic morning hike with Claudia Batten, who then became part of my team of expert readers, which also included Kristen D'Arcy and Anna Schecter. Their perspective proved invaluable when early drafts were a sprawl.

Endless gratitude to my sister and brother-in-law, Lauren and Christopher Loutit, for their steadfast moral support; to my beautiful sons, Will, George, and James, who are the lights and loves of my life; and to Michael Domitrovich and Keller and Jeff Fitzsimmons for spiritual guidance throughout.

Finally, I am beholden to my sources, including scientists who spent countless hours explaining knotty concepts and peeling back the veil on the scientific establishment. Most of all, I wish to thank Candace's family—especially Vanessa Pert, Evan Pert, Agu Pert, Nancy Glasser Morris, and Deane Beebe Fitzgerald—for their commitment to truth, and for walking with me on this long and painful road to discovery. The Rosenberg lineage is powerful and deeply loving, and I am forever grateful for their trust and faith in me.